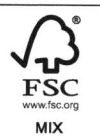

AF192149

Imprint

© 2025, copyright of the original edition of this
        book
© The text: Dr. Peter F. Mayer

Traude Schubert   traude-schubert@gmx.de

Cover image: https://www.piqsels.com/de/public-
domain-photo-fydpv

Publisher: BoD · Books on Demand GmbH,
In de Tarpen 42, 22848 Norderstedt, bod@bod.de
Print: Libri Plureos GmbH, Friedensallee 273,
22763 Hamburg
ISBN: 978-3-7693-5770-7

* * *

INFORMATION:

**We assume no guarantee and no liability for
the accuracy of the information provided in
this book.
It has been taken from the sources and
studies mentioned.
The translation was carried out with the help
of www.deeple.com .**

Traude Schubert
&
Dr. Peter F. Mayer
Publizist Science & Technology

MUSHROOMS

against cancer and

other diseases

Foreword by Traude Schubert

The word cancer gives almost everyone an uneasy feeling. That's what happened to me too. My mother had skin cancer.

Apart from chemotherapy, radiation and a few herbal preparations, there is hardly any help available.

But it does exist! I found out about this when I looked around in alternative media.

I found reports by Dr. Peter F. Mayer. He wrote about mushrooms that can demonstrably help with cancer!! What shocked me is that this has been known in Europe for years!

Dr. Mayer lists many studies on this that were very successful!

I then got in touch with him to make all this knowledge about mushrooms that can help with cancer better known.
This is how this book came about, in which I was able to include the reports and studies mentioned.

Attached are links to Dr. Peter F. Mayer's homepage, as well as further links to the individual studies.

We wish all patients much success with the therapies mentioned!

Traude Schubert

THANK YOU SO MUCH

My very special thanks go to

Dr. Peter F. Mayer,
Publicist Science & Technology,
Owner and editor of tkp.at
Homepage: https://tkp.at/

for allowing me to compile his articles with scientific evidence for the effects of various medicinal mushrooms into a book.

* * *

Please support the work of journalists with a donation.

The operation of tkp.at, remuneration for the work of journalists, technology and whatever else is required are essentially financed by our readers.
Support independent journalism with a donation!

Thank you very much!

Bank transfer
IBAN: AT03 1500 0042 2103 0523
BIC: OBKLAT2L
in the name of Dr. Peter F. Mayer

Paypal:
Peter Mayer @tkpPeterMayer

With your support you help to ensure that critical
journalism is not silenced! Thank you very much!

Link to this page:
https://tkp.at/unterstuetzen/

50% of my fee from this book goes as a donation
to TKP.

INFORMATION:

**We make no warranty or accept any liability
for the accuracy of the statements made in
this book.**

Contents

8

Mushrooms

AGAINST CANCER
AND OTHER DISEASES

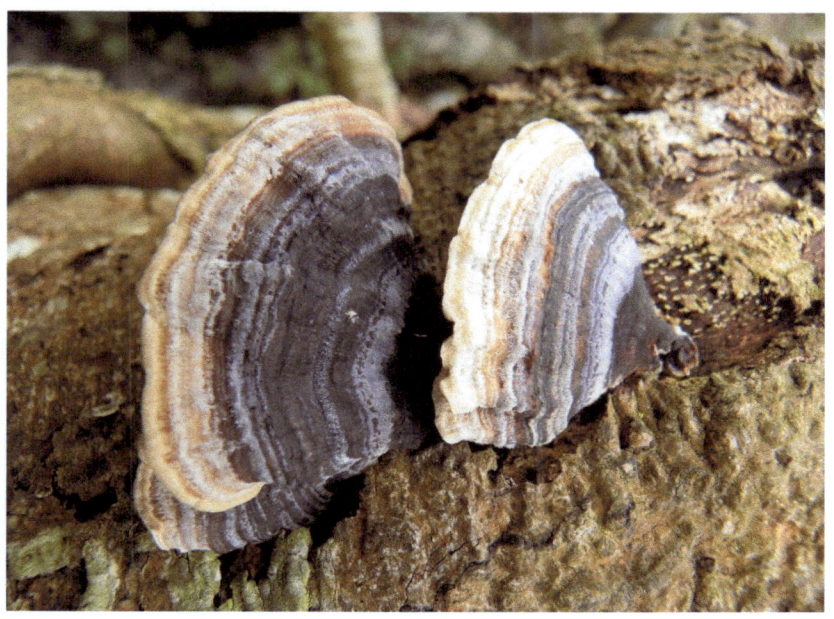

Huaeir Pilz

Cancer on the rise after vaccination - what helps against it

Link to this:
https://tkp.at/2024/04/20/krebs-nach-impfung-am-vormarsch-was-dagegen-hilft/
Author: Dr. Peter F. Mayer

For two years, it has become increasingly clear from the databases on side effects, mortality tables and anecdotal reports that the number of cancer cases has increased significantly worldwide since the vaccination campaign.
Even the WHO is expecting a massive increase in cancer cases, even if it sees the causes everywhere except in gene vaccination.

The question is, what can be done to prevent or treat it?
An mRNA vaccination against cancer?
Chemo?
Pfizer also expects a sharp increase in cancer cases to 30% of people and therefore last year acquired a company that has a new cancer drug for 43 billion dollars.

Link to this:
https://tkp.at/2023/03/14/turbokrebs-nach-mrna-impfung-pfizer-kauft-firma-mit-krebs-medikament-um-43-milliarden-dollar/

 You can read the entire report at this link or in my book "Our health is in grave danger! - Part 2" available soon.

Or should we do something else? And there are actually many options that we have reported on here on TKP time and again.

Let's take a look at what the experts have to say about it. The German Cancer Research Center (DKFZ) is particularly well-known and repeatedly points out that increasing vitamin D levels is an effective way to prevent cancer.

Link to this:
https://tkp.at/2021/02/13/deutsche-Krebsforscher-vitamin-d-schuetzt-vor-krebs-und-uebrigens-auch-vor-covid/
Please read the entire report on page 75,

In a press release published on February 11, 2021, it is reported that three meta-analyses of clinical studies in recent years have concluded that vitamin D supplementation was associated with a reduction in the death rate from cancer by around 13 percent.

Link to this:
https://www.dkfz.de/aktuelles/pressemitteilungen/detail/vitamin-d-supplementierung-moeglicher-gewinn-an-lebensjahren-bei-gleichzeitiger-kostenersparnis

Scientists at the DKFZ applied these results to the situation in Germany and calculated:
If all Germans over 50 were to receive vitamin D supplementation, up to 30,000 cancer deaths per year could be avoided and more than 300,000 years of life could be gained - while at the same time saving costs.

More in this TKP article.

Link to this:
https://tkp.at/2021/02/13/deutsche-krebsforscher-vitamin-d-schuetzt-vor-krebs-und-uebrigens-auch-vor-covid/
You can read the entire report on page 75.

This is not a particularly surprising finding, as it is clear that the immune system is the authority that destroys and eliminates tumor cells.

The 2018 Nobel Prize in Medicine went to researchers who showed that cancer can be best fought by strengthening the immune system.

It has to do with the HIF gene switch, which switches on genes for glycolysis and angiogenesis in the cancer cell. This allows the cancer to grow, feed itself and provide itself with blood. Oxygen and vitamin C are needed to break down HIF, because vitamin C is a co-factor of the enzyme that is crucial for the breakdown.

* * *

Vitamins and even more vitamins

Vitamin C is a powerful tool for fighting cancer. This was first demonstrated by the two-time Nobel Prize winner and chemist Linus Pauling, who suggested high doses of vitamin C for the treatment of cancer.
In studies, he and Ewan Cameron proved its effectiveness against cancer.

I would be happy to send you the PDF file.
Please write to: traude-schubert@gmx.de

This was verified in studies carried out by Creagan and Moertel at the Mayo Clinic. There was supposedly no advantage to administering high doses of vitamin C compared to administering a placebo.

However, the study was carried out incorrectly, the vitamin C was administered orally instead of as an infusion.

Professor Dr. Burkhard Kleuser, who studied chemistry and food chemistry from 1984 to 1988 and biochemistry from 1990 to 1994, and is therefore a natural scientist, explains in a longer article in the Pharmaceutical Journal the mode of action in the studies described by Linus Pauling:

Link to this:
https://www.pharmazeutische-zeitung.de/klassiker-im-neuen-licht/

"... it has been shown that oral administration of the most tolerable dose of 3 g every four hours leads to a maximum plasma concentration of 0.22 mmol/l.

In contrast, maximum plasma concentrations of more than 13 mmol/l were achieved when the vitamin C dose was administered intravenously. Similar results are also found in tumor patients."

* * *

We now come back to hydrogen peroxide:

"In high millimolar concentrations, which can only be achieved by intravenous administration, vitamin C acts as a prooxidant and leads to the formation of hydrogen peroxide, which is capable of damaging tumor cells."
In lower concentrations, vitamin C acts as a strong antioxidant, in high concentrations as a pro-oxidant. Only a small amount of hydrogen peroxide is produced. ... Only when vitamin C passes from the bloodstream into the interstitium [connective tissue] does an intensive formation of hydrogen peroxide occur, which can then selectively damage tumor cells as a cytotoxic molecule... .

The effect seems to be specific to tumor cells because, in contrast to healthy cells, these often have little or no activity of antioxidant enzymes such as catalase, glutathione peroxidase and superoxide dismutase, which would be able to break down hydrogen peroxide.
We see once again that the dose makes the poison. "As long as the vitamin C circulates in the blood, it will detoxify."

The orthomolecular physician and author Dr. Ulrich Strunz describes in his blog about cancer treatment and the experiences of a patient with oncologists:

"And she is told by her oncologist: Please no vitamin C infusion.
This "disturbs" the chemotherapy treatment."

Link to this:
https://www.drstrunz.de/aktuelles/2021/11/20211108_Vitamin_C_stoert_Chemotherapie.php

And further:
"Let's use our brains for a moment and be sensible:

- Vitamin C has a half-life in the blood of 2.9 hours. So if you get vitamin C infusions today and chemotherapy tomorrow, so the whole thing is delayed, then the chemotherapy won't notice the vitamin C at all.
- This is called simple natural science. I emphasize the word "simple!".
- Much more important is the following consideration:
- How does chemotherapy work? This poison generates massive amounts of free radicals in every cell in the body. And hopefully more free radicals in the cancer cell, which has a higher metabolic rate, than in the healthy cells. Agreed. Free radicals in this concentration destroy, kill cells.
- Both: cancer cells and healthy cells. Hopefully the cancer died sooner than the patient. I mean that in a very decent and respectful way. I have often given such infusions myself...
- How do vitamin C infusions work? Vitamin C in this high dose (and only then) produces massive

amounts of H_2O_2, i.e. hydrogen peroxide, a strong cell poison, a free radical in every cell.
But healthy cells still have the enzyme catalase. And it breaks down this H_2O_2, these free radicals, at lightning speed.
The poor cancer cell is at a disadvantage:
It no longer has any catalase, is defenseless against the poison. It dies."

Exciting.
Vitamin C acts on the one hand as an antioxidant, catching free radicals, and on the other hand as a pro-oxidant, producing $H2O2$ in the body, which is able to oxidize tumor cells and thus eliminate them. In the article, Kleuser lists other ways in which vitamin C works against tumors.

He mentions that

"Vitamin C also plays a central role in the regulation of »Ten-Eleven-Translocation« (TET) enzymes and »Jumonji domain-containing histone« demethylases."

"Another way in which vitamin C can have an effect on tumor cells is through the modulation of the hypoxia-induced factor HIF. …. the expression of the vascular endothelial growth factor VEGF occurs, which promotes angiogenesis and thus the blood supply to the tumor."

* * *

Mushrooms and oxygen

Japanese studies have shown that Huaier mushrooms (Trametes robiniophila murr) not only cure cancer up to stage IV, but also remove vaccine spikes from the body.

Link to this:
https://tkp.at/2023/05/30/japanische-studie-zeigt-wie-huaier-pilz-krebs-bekaempft-und-schaedliche-impf-spike-aus-dem-koerper-entfernt/
You can read the full report on page 33.

This is also a prerequisite for curing mRNA-induced cancer.
There are detailed TKP articles about this here and here.

Links to this:
https://tkp.at/2022/10/05/studie-c19-impfungen-fuehren-zu-vorzeitiger-zell-alterung-und-foerdern-krebserkrankung-video-mit-florian-schilling/
You can read the full report on page 42.

https://tkp.at/2023/05/30/japanische-studie-zeigt-wie-huaier-pilz-krebs-bekaempft-und-schaedliche-impf-spike-aus-dem-koerper-entfernt/
You can read the full report on page 33.

Other mushrooms have long been said to have similar effects on cancer, such as the Chaga mushroom, which has a strong regulating and strengthening effect on the immune system.
Something similar can be achieved with the butterfly mushroom.

Let's move on to oxygen.

We have known for about 100 years that tumor cells feed on sugar by fermenting it, i.e. without oxygen.
This discovery comes from the German biochemist Professor Otto Warburg (Nobel Prize 1931). Warburg was able to show that cancer cells live primarily on sugar and ferment it without oxygen - even though there is enough oxygen available. With a rather poor energy yield.

At the University of Graz, Professor Frank Madeo was able to show that
> • reducing cell respiration (i.e. shortness of breath) reduces programmed, natural cell death, known as apoptosis, and therefore cells live uncontrollably.

> • Uncontrolled survival means rapid growth, which means cancer.

Link to this:
https://tkp.at/2022/06/17/masken-koennten-das-wachstum-von-krebs-foerdern/
You can read the entire report on page 81.

Prof. Madeo: "This increased resistance (to cell death) could make a decisive contribution to tumor formation and malignancy (metastasis)."
The study entitled "The Warburg Effect Suppresses Oxidative Stress Induced Apoptosis in a Yeast Model for Cancer"

Link to this:

https://journals.plos.org/plosone/article?id=10.1371/journal.pone.0004592

(The Warburg effect suppresses apoptosis triggered by oxidative stress in a yeast model for cancer) was published in Plos One.
With this model, the Graz researchers were able to prove that cells have a survival advantage through the so-called Warburg effect.

So

- aggressive cancer cells feed on sugar (glycolysis)
- while simultaneously reducing oxygen respiration.

Increased respiratory activity, i.e. more oxygen supply, inhibits the growth of tumors. According to Madeo.
The slim university professor goes on to explain:
"Interestingly, endurance sports are one of the best preventive measures against cancer. This increases the body's oxygen supply and also consumes sugar. Both, according to the classic Warburg hypothesis, are poison for the cancer cell."

The conclusion of the study is:

"The Warburg effect could therefore contribute directly to the development of cancer - not only through increased glycolysis, but also through reduced respiration in the presence of oxygen, which suppresses apoptosis."

Accordingly, radioactively labeled sugar and oxygen isotopes are used to diagnose cancer.

Where there is a lot of sugar, there is a tumor.

Where there is little oxygen, the tumor develops.
The treatment is to do the opposite of the diagnosis:
Little or no sugar (and carbohydrates) and lots of oxygen, says Dr. Ulrich Strunz and anyone who can think logically.

* * *

Cancer treatment highly effective with Chaga medicinal mushroom - studies

Link to this:
https://tkp.at/2024/05/01/krebs-behandlung-hochwirksam-mit-chaga-heilpilz-studien/
Author: Dr. Peter F. Mayer

The number of cancer cases has increased rapidly in the past three years and continues to grow. This raises the question of efficient treatments and preventative measures. In addition to chemotherapy, which has serious side effects, biochemistry has natural methods to offer.
Medicinal mushrooms offer other highly effective approaches, as studies have shown several times.

I recently gave an overview of the various options for effectively fighting cancer in this article.

Link to this:
https://tkp.at/2024/04/20/krebs-nach-impfung-am-vormarsch-was-dagegen-hilft/
You can read the entire report on this on page 12 in this book.

It also mentions the Chaga medicinal mushroom, but without citing any studies on it. I would like to make up for that here. Chaga is highly effective against cancer and has a whole range of effects that support and regulate the immune system.

This has already been proven in many studies.
Here are two of them.

First, here is a quote from one study:

"The extract of I. obliquus had a significant
tumor-suppressive effect in both models. In
mice that had a tumor, **a 60 percent
reduction in the tumor was observed**, while
in mice with **metastases the number of
nodes decreased by 25% compared to the
control group.**

In addition, the mice treated with I.
obliquus extract showed an increase in tumor
agglomeration and an inhibition of
vascularization.   Interestingly, taking I.
obliquus reduced the body weight of middle-
aged mice and increased body temperature in
response to the light-dark cycle in adult mice.
In addition, I. obliquus prevented a drop in
temperature in mice after tumor implantation."

**The result was achieved after just three weeks of
taking Chaga extracts:**

"The anti-cancer effect of I. obliquus extract
was investigated in mouse models for the
growth of Lewis lung carcinoma and
spontaneous metastasis after three weeks of
continuous intake of the extract at a dose of 6
mg/kg/day, which corresponds to the daily
intake of Chaga infusions in Japan."

The study by Satoru Arata et al entitled "Continuous intake of the Chaga mushroom (Inonotus obliquus) aqueous extract suppresses cancer progression and maintains body temperature in mice"

Link to this:
https://pmc.ncbi.nlm.nih.gov/articles/PMC4946216/

(The continuous intake of the aqueous extract of the Chaga mushroom (Inonotus obliquus) suppresses the progression of cancer and maintains body temperature in mice) was published in May 2016.

The Chaga mushroom - Inonotus obliquus or slate slate polypore - grows in the far north and is said to be more effective the further north it grows. It is mainly available in Scandinavian or Baltic countries.
It is available as a fine powder, in capsules or as chunks (picture above) for making tea.
There are a number of companies that sell medicinal and vital mushrooms of high organic quality.

* * *

The study explains its occurrence:

"Medicinal mushrooms have long been used in traditional oriental therapy and as nutritional foods.

Inonotus obliquus (Chaga mushroom), which belongs to the Hymenochaetaceae family of basidiomycetes, grows primarily on the trunks of mature, living birch trees.

The basic effect of Chaga is to strengthen and regulate the immune system.
Regulatory in the sense that malfunctions, for example in autoimmune diseases, are dampened or switched off.

* * *

The study on effects (see references):

Link here:
https://pmc.ncbi.nlm.nih.gov/articles/PMC4946216/

"The extracts of I. obliquus are used in China, Korea, Japan, Russia and the Baltic States for their beneficial effects on lipid metabolism and heart function as well as for their antibacterial, anti-inflammatory, antioxidant and anti-tumor effects. Extracts of I. obliquus were found to inhibit hepatitis C virus [10] and human immunodeficiency virus [11, 12] and exhibit potent antioxidant and immunostimulatory effects in vitro [13, 14]

At the same time, animal studies showed that aqueous extracts of I. obliquus exhibited anti-inflammatory effects in experimental colitis [15, 16] and promoted lipid metabolism [17]. Several studies investigated the anti-tumor activity of the aqueous extract of I. obliquus and found that it suppressed the proliferation [18] of various carcinoma cell lines and induced apoptosis [19].

In addition, the compounds isolated from I. obliquus extracts have been shown to inhibit skin carcinogenesis [20] and tumor growth in mice bearing sarcoma 180 cells [21]."

* * *

Here are 11 of 30 other studies that show very positive and beneficial effects of Chaga.

Study on the effect of Chaga on bladder cancer

Die Studie von Amira Abugomaa et al mit dem Titel „*Anti-cancer activity of Chaga mushroom (Inonotus obliquus) against dog bladder cancer organoids*" (Anti-cancer activity of the Chaga mushroom (Inonotus obliquus) against organoids of dog bladder cancer) is more recent, was published on 19 April 2023.

Link to this:
https://www.frontiersin.org/journals/pharmacology/articles/10.3389/fphar.2023.1159516/full

* * *

First, the problem of the classical therapeutic approaches is described:

"To date, the first-line treatment of MIBC is radical cystectomy (transurethral resection) followed by adjuvant chemoradiotherapy (Knapp et al., 2014; Fulkerson and Knapp, 2015).

27

However, the side effects and the development of resistance to chemotherapy are the main problems leading to treatment failure and recurrence of BC.
Therefore, the introduction of new adjunctive herbal therapies with anti-cancer properties can provide synergistic effects and reduce the side effects associated with chemotherapy, which will be of great benefit to cancer patients."

* * *

And here is a brief summary of what the Chaga mushroom does and against which types of cancer it has been tested in studies:

"Chaga mushrooms (Inonotus obliquus) are a whitish mushroom that belongs to the Hymenochaetaceae family and grows on birch roots in several countries (Lee et al., 2008).

Link to this:
https://www.frontiersin.org/journals/pharmacol ogy/articles/10.3389/fphar.2023.1159516/ full#B23

Chaga mushrooms are said to have various health-promoting effects, including antimicrobial, anti-inflammatory, antioxidant and antitumor effects (Balandaykin and Zmitrovich, 2015).

28

Link to this:
https://www.frontiersin.org/journals/pharmacology/articles/10.3389/fphar.2023.1159516/full#B23

Therefore, Chaga mushroom extract (Chaga) is used as a traditional medicine in Asia and Eastern Europe (Balandaykin and Zmitrovich, 2015).

Link to this:
https://www.frontiersin.org/journals/pharmacology/articles/10.3389/fphar.2023.1159516/full#B6

Recently, several reports have shown that Chaga has cytotoxic effects against various types of cancer cells such as sarcoma (Chung et al., 2010), lung adenocarcinoma (Baek et al., 2018), colon cancer (Lee et al., 2009), melanoma (Youn et al., 2009) and hepatocellular carcinoma (Youn et al., 2008). Therefore, Chaga is often consumed by cancer patients as an herbal supplement (Buckner et al., 2018)."

Links to this:
https://www.frontiersin.org/journals/pharmacology/articles/10.3389/fphar.2023.1159516/full#B8

https://www.frontiersin.org/journals/pharma-cology/articles/10.3389/fphar.2023.1159516/full#B5

https://www.frontiersin.org/journals/pharmacology/articles/10.3389/fphar.2023.1159516/full#B24

https://www.frontiersin.org/journals/pharmacology/articles/10.3389/fphar.2023.1159516/full#B43

https://www.frontiersin.org/journals/pharmacology/articles/10.3389/fphar.2023.1159516/full#B42

https://www.frontiersin.org/journals/pharmacology/articles/10.3389/fphar.2023.1159516/full#B7

* * *

So we see that the spectrum of effects of Chaga is very broad and has been demonstrated for a whole range of cancer types.

The results of the study itself are summarized as follows:

In summary, we have investigated the antitumor potential of Chaga on DBCO for the first time.

Chaga inhibits DBCO by stopping the cell cycle, triggering apoptosis, reducing the state of stem cells and thus impairing cell proliferation (Figure 9).

Chaga has also been found to enhance the effects of common cancer drugs used for BC therapy.   30

Studies on medicinal mushrooms in connection with corona vaccinations

Japanese studies have shown that Huaier mushrooms (Trametes robiniophila murr) not only cure cancer up to stage IV, but also remove vaccination spikes from the body. This is also a prerequisite for curing mRNA-induced cancer.

Link to this:
https://tkp.at/2023/05/30/japanische-studie-zeigt-wie-huaier-pilz-krebs-bekaempft-und-schaedliche-impf-spike-aus-dem-koerper-entfernt/
You can read the full report on page 33 in this book.

There are detailed TKP articles about this here and here. Chaga is likely to have similar effects to Huaier.

Link to this:
https://tkp.at/2022/10/05/studie-c19-impfungen-fuehren-zu-vorzeitiger-zell-alterung-und-foerdern-krebserkrankung-video-mit-florian-schilling/
You can read the full report on page 42 in this book.

The researchers led by Manami Tanaka et al conducted a study entitled 'Huaier Effects on Functional Compensation with Destructive Ribosomal RNA Structure after Anti-SARS-CoV-2 mRNA Vaccination', in which they administered Huaier mushrooms to cancer patients.

Link to this:

https://www.fortunejournals.com/articles/huaier-effects-on-functional-compensation-with-destructive-ribosomal-rna-structure-after-antisarscov2-mrna-vaccination.html

The fungus, which is unfortunately not yet directly available in Europe but according to TKP readers could be delivered to resellers by Chinese mail order companies, but this fails due to the lack of EU approval, even cures types of cancer such as pancreatic or colon cancer, both of which are among the more deadly.

Note from me:
Currently no longer available!
However, German pharmacies and natural medicine distributors now also sell Huaier powder.

However, a vaccination immediately brings the cancer back to life and leads to death, as the study shows. However, the fungus still protects.

The follow-up study is entitled "Huaier Effects on Prevention and Inhibition of Spontaneous SARS-CoV-2 Virion Production by Repeated Pfizer-BioNTech mRNA Vaccination" and is concerned with further elucidating the damaging mechanisms of the vaccination spike and how the protection provided by the fungi works.

Link to this:

https://www.fortunejournals.com/articles/huaier-effects-on-prevention-and-inhibition-of-spontaneous-sarscov2-virion-production-by-repeated-pfizerbiontech-mrna-vaccination.html

Japanese study shows how Huaier mushroom fights cancer and removes harmful vaccine spikes from the body

Link to this:
https://tkp.at/2023/05/30/japanische-studie-zeigt-wie-huaier-pilz-krebs-bekaempft-und-schaedliche-impf-spike-aus-dem-koerper-entfernt/
Author: Dr. Peter F. Mayer

Study: C19 vaccinations lead to premature cell aging and promote cancer - video with Florian Schilling
Shedding (transmission) of corona vaccination spikes confirmed again by study.
This is how you can deactivate spikes in the body!

Link to this:
https://tkp.at/2024/12/18/tcm-medikament-huaier-pilz-laut-studien-hochwirksam-gegen-krebs-und-impfschaeden/
You can read the complete report on page 62!

Last year, TKP reported here on a sensational Japanese study that looked at the cure of stage four cancer by administering Huaier.
Apparently by chance, it turned out that Huaier also protects against damage caused by vaccination spikes and can remove them from the body even after multiple vaccinations.

There is now a very interesting follow-up study on this.

Doctors have used the article and the explanatory video by the incomparable Florian Schilling as an opportunity to use fungal therapy to combat the negative effects of vaccination and remove spikes from the body.
The problem with Huaier is that you can't get it in Europe.

Note from me:
In the meantime, some pharmacies and natural medicine companies have Huaier mushrooms on offer as powder.

For example here:
https://nutrimentas-shop.de/products/vitalpilz-huaier-trametes-robiniophila-fur-forschunge-wecke

* * *

The scientific name of Huaier is Trametes robiniophila murr.

There are a lot of Trametes here and it has been shown that the hirsuta (Trametes hirsuta - picture above) has the same effects and removes spikes from the body as effectively as the Huaier mushroom.

If you would like to know more about the cancer effects of Huaier, you can get the book by the two study authors Manami Tanaka and Tomoo Tanaka:

Link to this:

The description states:

This book explains why and how Huaier can treat and cure the various types of cancer, even in advanced stages, without any toxicity or side effects.

A comprehensive genetic analysis has revealed the molecular basis of Huaier's anti-cancer effect:

1) Promoting cancer-specific cell death within the pathogenic lesion;

2) Clearing the resulting damaged cell debris;

3) Restoring damaged and/or dissected tissue with normal cells (tissue regeneration; transcriptional regulation of pluripotency in induced pluripotent stem cells (iPS)/embryonic stem cells (ES));

4) Preventing relapses and recurrences, as well as adjacent and extensive metastases.

The effect of Huaier against cancer and vaccination spikes

The first study involved 8 people whose stage 4 cancer had been cured by Huaier.
The vaccination caused the cancer to flare up again and die within a very short time in the participants who did not take the Huaier.
There were no changes and no problems in the patients who continued taking Huaier.

The researchers located the problems with serial vaccinations in the destructive effects on the molecular mechanisms of protein synthesis through the destruction of ribosomal RNA structures.
In these central structures of the cell, the ribosomes, the enzymes are produced without which no life is possible.
Their destruction or disability leads to death.
Before this study, no one had realized that the vaccine damage occurs through the penetration of the spike into this deepest level of the cells.

The follow-up study is entitled 'Huaier Effects on Prevention and Inhibition of Spontaneous SARS-CoV-2 Virion Production by Repeated Pfizer-BioNTech mRNA Vaccination' and deals with the further elucidation of the damaging mechanisms of the vaccination spike and how the
by Repeated Pfizer-BioNTech mRNA Vaccination) and deals with the further elucidation of the damaging mechanisms of the vaccination spike and how the protection by the fungi works.

"As part of our clinical research, we observed and reported spontaneous production of SARS-CoV-2 virions and virion parts after the Pfizer-BioNTech mRNA vaccination, which occurred starting 3 weeks after the first injection.

Significant destruction of ribosomal RNA structures was also observed, which was enhanced by repeated vaccinations.
The aim of the present study is to define the molecular mechanisms for the production of SARS-CoV-2 virions after injection of mRNA vaccination and to compare them with virion propagation in unvaccinated patients with severe COVID-19 pneumonia and fibrosis."

* * *

The methods are described:

"We are conducting clinical research to define the molecular basis for the significant anti-cancer efficacy of Huaier (Trametes robiniophila murr).

In the present study, we used peripheral blood samples from volunteer patients with suspected lung cancer by CT image analysis and age-matched normal controls with or without Huaier administration.

Molecular characterization was performed by sequencing total RNA and non-coding small RNA on the BGISEQ-500 platform (approximately 7.0 GB analysis per sample)."

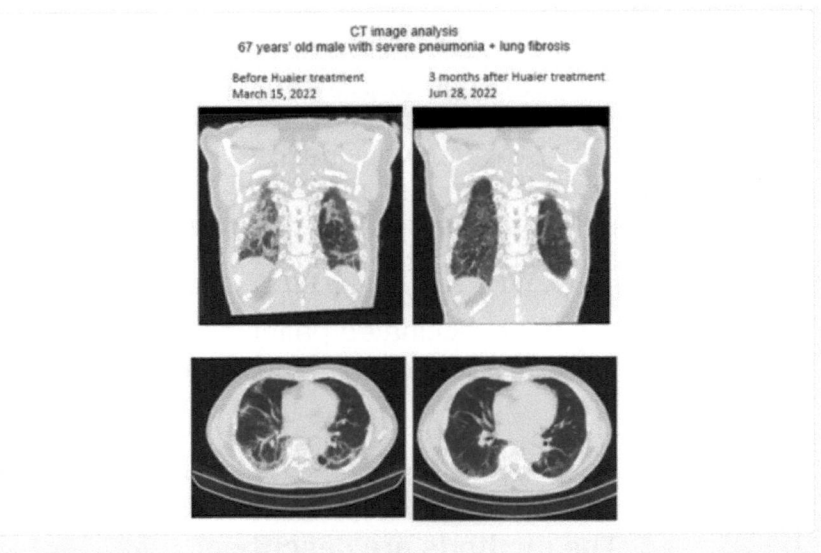

Figure 1: Chest CT image analysis before (March 15) and after 3 months of Huaier treatment on the patient (June 28).

* * *

Regarding the effect on the vaccination spike, the researchers write:

"Normal individuals can usually eliminate foreign genetic material within a few days, but production of SARS-CoV-2 in vivo was detected starting three weeks after the first vaccination and continued even five months after the third vaccination.

The influence of injected self-replicating mRNAs, in addition to subsequent spontaneous production, remains unclear.

In addition, even with multiple vaccinations, there is still the possibility of COVID-19 infection with new mutated strains.

The preventive efficacy of repeated vaccinations against SARS-CoV-2 is limited, and most importantly, problems with serial vaccination have been raised regarding the destructive effects on the molecular mechanisms of protein synthesis by destroying ribosomal RNA structures. …

We found that Huaier can compensate for any damage caused by destructive ribosomal RNA structures after mRNA vaccination against SARS-CoV-2, depending on the genomic potential of each individual, regardless of the severity of cancer or basic health conditions.

An accelerated aging process in lipid metabolism was also observed, which affects the production of microemboli and leads to an increasing number of brain and heart attacks in the Japanese population.

In the present study, together with the previous report, we managed to find a clue and a solution to these problems, including a strategy for prevention and treatment without any complications.

It is also pointed out that the repair of destroyed ribosomal RNA structures was a good indicator of the risk of spontaneous virion production as well as a good indicator of the recovery process.

The molecular systems responsible for these improvements were closely related to the aging process via the activation of mTOR/PI3K/AKT kinase-related signaling networks, as previously reported. ....

A low dose of Huaier, 6 g per day, is sufficient to prevent SARS-CoV-2 infection as well as unexpected damage in molecular systems under these normal controls.

Huaier effects contributed to the regulation of kinase functions via mTOR/PI3K/AKT signaling networks, which cooperated with massive mi- and pi-RNA-driven transcriptional control.

The present study thus provides an efficient and safe strategy to cope with the upcoming post-pandemic COVID-19 era."

The authors also report that the Pfizer-BioNTech and Moderna vaccines, when injected, deliver the mRNA to the cells, which not only produce copies of the of the expected spike, but also promote spontaneous virion production.

But administration of Huaier resulted in a significant downregulation of these virions and particles derived from them, which was not dependent on the Huaier dose.

One study participant in the untreated control group opted to receive Huaier (20 g per day) three weeks after the fourth vaccination.

The researchers expect the damaged ribosomal RNA structure to be restored and changed, as massive hair growth was observed within a month of Huaier treatment.

From what I have received feedback, **Bristly Tramete** should have similar effects to the vaccine spikes as Huaier.

* * *

Cancer therapies with mushrooms are also common in Europe.

There are reports of successful applications, for example with the **butterfly tramete** (Trametes versicolor, also Coriolus versicolor) or in northern countries with the Chaga mushroom.

The study is relatively easy to read, it is worth going t**o the original.**
The study population is small, but causalities are investigated using scientific methods and not just any correlations.

Link to the original study:
https://www.fortunejournals.com/articles/huaier-effects-on-prevention-and-inhibition-of-spontaneous-sarscov2-virion-production-by-repeated-pfizerbiontech-mrna-vaccination.html

* * *

Study: C19 vaccinations lead to premature cell aging and promote cancer -

Video with Florian Schilling

Links to this:

https://tkp.at/2022/10/05/studie-c19-impfungen-fuehren-zu-vorzeitiger-zell-alterung-und-foerdern-krebserkrankung-video-mit-florian-schilling/

Author: Dr. Peter F. Mayer

A new study shows that the vaccination disrupts or destroys the ribosomes and thus the metabolism. Cell aging, multimorbidity and diseases are the result. Conversely, an overfunction of malignant cells is caused. A fungus can, however, compensate for the harmful effects of the vaccination.

The damage to the ribosomes explains the excess mortality and premature, unexplained deaths. Florian Schilling explains in detail how and why this happens in the video below.

The researchers led by Manami Tanaka et al conducted a study entitled 'Huaier Effects on Functional Compensation with Destructive Ribosomal RNA Structure after Anti-SARS-CoV-2 mRNA Vaccination'. (Huaier Effects on Functional Compensation with Destructive Ribosomal RNA Structure after Anti-SARS-CoV-2 mRNA Vaccination), in which they administered Huaier mushrooms to cancer patients.

Link to this:
https://www.fortunejournals.com/articles/huaier-effects-on-functional-compensation-with-destructive-ribosomal-rna-structure-after-antisarscov2-mrna-vaccination.html

The therapy comes from Chinese medicine. A very well-conducted study, albeit with a very small cohort of 8 patients.
However, very clear differences can be seen.

The methodology of the study consists of RNA sequencing. This shows which genes are active and what has changed as a result of the vaccination.
The most important finding is that the vaccination destroys the ribosomes and therefore various signaling pathways in the cell are massively weakened.
The damage was more persistent and massive than after chemotherapy and increased with each subsequent injection.

The bottom line is premature aging, premature multimorbidity.
The destruction of the ribosomes is so critically harmful because they are the protein factories of the cells. They produce enzymes, for example - and without them there is no metabolism, the cell dies and the body dies.

The fungus even cures types of cancer such as pancreatic or colon cancer, both of which are among the more deadly.

A vaccination, however, immediately brings the cancer

back to life and leads to death, as the study shows.
The fungus can, however, protect.

The abstract of the study states, among other things:

We analyzed biological changes by sequencing total RNA in healthy volunteers and cancer patients vaccinated by Pfizer-BioNTech, with or without adjuvant Huaier therapy.

Significant destruction of ribosomal RNA structures was observed, which was enhanced by serial vaccinations. In contrast to destruction by platinum(II) complex chemotherapy, progressive destruction of the 18S ribosome was observed even 6 months after vaccination. This led to massive inhibition of translation and transcription, which had a significant impact on intra-/internal neuronal signaling and lipid metabolism and was related to the aging process.

Huaier compensated for these dysfunctions through miRNA-mediated transcriptional control, namely through typical activation of the PI3K/AKT signaling pathway.

The Gene Ontology analysis showed that the number of virions was still produced spontaneously 3 months after the first vaccination.
The present study shows that adjuvant therapy such as Huaier compensates for the accelerated aging process caused by the mRNA vaccination.

Link to the video:
https://rumble.com/v1lz050-bad-news-from-japan.html

Butterfly Tramete helps against cancer - studies

Source:
https://tkp.at/2024/05/08/schmetterlings-tramete-hilft-gegen-krebs-studien/
Report by Dr. Peter F. Mayer

One consequence of the Corona mRNA vaccination campaign is the sharp increase in the number of cancer cases.
In order to drive out the devil with Beelzebub, the pharmaceutical industry is relying on more genetic engineering with mRNA anti-cancer preparations. However, there are a number of natural healing and treatment methods, including medicinal mushrooms such as the butterfly tramete.

I recently presented studies in which the effectiveness of the **Chaga mushroom** against cancer was investigated. I have presented other effective treatment and healing methods in this article.

Japanese studies have shown that Huaier mushrooms (Trametes robiniophila murr) not only cure cancer up to stage IV, but also remove vaccine spikes from the body.

This is also a prerequisite for curing mRNA-induced cancer. There are detailed TKP articles about this here and here = see the following article!

Trametes are native to practically every country, and at least 40 different species can be found in the forests of Central Europe.
And if you search the internet for the terms "vital mushroom" or "medicinal mushroom", you will find a number of suppliers who can offer various preparations.

If you search the medical database Pubmed for the butterfly tramete with its scientific name Trametes versicolor (Synn. Coriolus versicolor – CV), you will get 1192 hits; if you also restrict the search to cancer, you will get 50 results.

Number 1 on the list of finds is Habtemariam S. with *"Trametes versicolor (Synn. Coriolus versicolor) Polysaccharides in Cancer Therapy: Targets and Efficacy".*
The study provides an overview of the effects and mechanisms of action regarding direct cytotoxicity in cancer cells and the immune-stimulating effect.

* * *

The conclusions describe the results from hundreds of other studies:

"... Polysaccharide peptide (PSP) and polysaccharide K (PSK, Krestin) as well as other polysaccharides from C. versicolor have also been shown to induce direct cytotoxicity for cancer/tumor cells.
They also increase the release of cytokines such as TNF-α, which is directly linked to the killing of tumor cells.

The general anti-cancer pharmacology of these polysaccharides through a direct effect on cancer cells and an indirect effect via immune stimulation is shown in Figure 3.

Overall, the polysaccharides of C. versicolor have been shown to directly inhibit cell growth and induce apoptosis in cancer cells.
In some cases, cell cycle arrest was observed even at concentrations less than 100 µg/mL in vitro.
This modest level of activity should be considered significant since the active components are high molecular weight compounds or mixtures.
Since orally ingested carbohydrates are hydrolyzed by intestinal enzymes, the question always arises as to whether they can retain their therapeutic value in vivo. Interestingly, C. versicolor polysaccharides, including PSP and PSK, have shown anticancer activity in vivo following oral administration.

Another known mechanism for the anticancer effect of C. versicolor is its immunostimulatory effect, as evidenced by the ability of the polysaccharides to increase the production of cytokines such as IL-12, which is associated with Th1. Th lymphocyte subsets, including Th1, Th2, Th17 or Treg, mainly through the production of key cytokines and lymphocyte subsets (B cells, CD4+ and CD8+ T cells, NK cells and different stages of differentiated T cells) have been extensively studied for their response to C. versicolor polysaccharides.

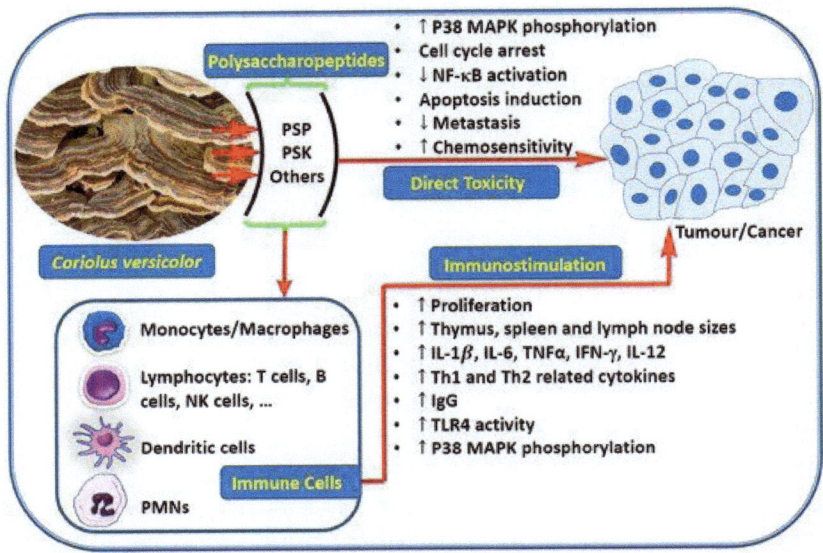

Figure 3.
Anticancer potential of C. versivolor polysaccharides.

It has been shown that cytokines such as IFN-γ are induced in T cells, which together with TNF-α cause the killing of cancer/tumors.
Other cytokines, including IL-1 and IL-6, have been shown to be enhanced by the polysaccharides.
All of these events appear to increase antibody production in T cells while simultaneously increasing the activity of other mononuclear cells, including monocytes/macrophages."

The mechanisms of action are apparently already relatively well understood.
These are natural biochemical reactions of the immune system that are elicited or enhanced.

48

Some studies also look at how the butterfly tramete can be used to reduce side effects of classic chemotherapy and radiotherapy and make the therapy effective.
There are also a number of articles in which the effects of Coriolus on various types of cancer have been investigated.

An interesting paper looks at the benefits of tramete for Covid-19 and cancer.

* * *

The strong anti-cancer effects of mushrooms

Article on this topic:
https://tkp.at/2025/02/09/die-starken-anti-krebs-wirkungen-von-pilzen/
Author: Dr. Peter F. Mayer

The scientific evidence for the health effects of mushrooms is numerous.
The mechanisms of action have also been well researched. In addition, they have been important remedies in Chinese medicine and natural medicine worldwide for thousands of years. Especially now, with the increased incidence of cancer and turbo cancer caused by the corona vaccination campaign, they have many areas of application.

TKP has been reporting for several years on studies that have shown high effectiveness against all types of cancer in various medicinal mushrooms.
The McCullough Foundation has now also taken up the topic of mushrooms and Nicolas Hulscher gives an overview of the effects of Huaier, butterfly bracket fungus, Chaga and some other mushrooms.

Link to this:
https://petermcculloughmd.substack.com/p/the-remarkable-anti-cancer-potential?utm_source=post-email-title&publication_id=1119676&post_id=156696812&utm_campaign=email-post-title&isFreemail=false&r=8sqvf&triedRedirect=true&utm_medium=email

He summarizes scientific evidence and practical experience and points out that biological mechanisms, epidemiological evidence and clinical data support the use of mushrooms in cancer prevention and treatment.

He reports that the health freedom movement is tired of experimental gene therapies and is looking for safer, more natural approaches to cancer prevention and treatment.
This is also our experience with feedback from our readers.
Dr. John Catanzaro, founder of Neo7Bioscience, has demonstrated the potential of precision engineered peptides and small molecules for personalized cancer treatment.

Link here:
https://johncatanzaro.substack.com/cp/156522429

Dr. William Makis and many others are advocating for the use of ivermectin and fenbendazole in cancer treatment, which has shown great promise.

Link here:
https://www.youtube.com/watch?v=0gIYQCjB_NU
The video is in English!

Another promising but often overlooked approach in Western medicine is the use **of mushrooms in cancer.** Hulscher summarizes the biological mechanisms, epidemiological evidence and clinical data that support the use of mushrooms in cancer prevention and treatment.

Biological mechanisms

Pathak et al. (Immunomodulatory effect of mushrooms and their bioactive compounds in cancer: A comprehensive review) investigated the immunomodulatory effect of mushrooms and their bioactive compounds in cancer:

Link to this:
https://www.sciencedirect.com/science/article/pii/S0753332222002906#bib141

- **Immunomodulation**:
Bioactive compounds in mushrooms such as lentinan, schizophyllan and maitake D fraction stimulate the immune system by activating macrophages, dendritic cells and natural killer cells (NK cells), thereby increasing cytokine production (e.g. IL-2, IL-6, TNF-α) and enhancing the immune response against tumors.

- **Cell cycle arrest:**
Polysaccharides and other phytochemicals in mushrooms can stop cancer cell division at key regulatory checkpoints, especially in the G0/G1 and G2/M phases, thereby preventing tumor proliferation.

- **Apoptosis induction:** Fungi trigger programmed cell death (apoptosis) in cancer cells via both the intrinsic (mitochondrial) and extrinsic (death receptor) pathways, leading to DNA fragmentation and caspase activation, effectively eliminating malignant cells.

• **Inhibition of angiogenesis:**
Certain fungi, such as Ganoderma lucidum and Phellinus linteus, block the formation of new blood vessels (angiogenesis) that tumors need for growth by downregulating vascular endothelial growth factor (VEGF) and inhibiting endothelial cell proliferation.

• **Regulation of oxidative stress:**
Fungal compounds such as ergothioneine, glutathione, and polyphenols neutralize reactive oxygen species (ROS), thereby reducing oxidative DNA damage that contributes to carcinogenesis.

* * *

Epidemiological evidence

Ba et al. (Higher Mushroom Consumption Is Associated with Lower Risk of Cancer: A Systematic Review and Meta-Analysis of Observational Studies) conducted a systematic review and meta-analysis of observational studies examining the association between mushroom consumption and cancer risk and found a significant inverse relationship:

Link here:
https://pmc.ncbi.nlm.nih.gov/articles/PMC8483951/

• **Reduction in overall cancer risk:**
Higher mushroom consumption was associated with a 34% lower risk of overall cancer (pooled RR: 0.66; 95% CI: 0.55–0.78; n = 17 studies).

• **Reduction in breast cancer risk:**
The strongest association was seen for breast cancer, with a 35% lower risk in the group with the highest mushroom consumption (pooled RR: 0.65; 95% CI: 0.52–0.81; n = 10 studies).

• **Reduction in risk of cancers other than breast cancer:**
A smaller reduction in other cancers was seen (pooled RR: 0.80; 95% CI: 0.66–0.97; n = 13 studies).

• **Dose-response relationship:**
A nonlinear dose-response relationship was seen (P = 0.001), showing a 45% lower risk with mushroom intake of 18 g/day compared to 0 g/day.

* * *

Clinical data

Narayanan et al. (Medicinal Mushroom Supplements in Cancer: A Systematic Review of Clinical Studies) conducted a systematic review of clinical trials examining the use of medicinal mushrooms in cancer treatment and found evidence of potential benefits in terms of survival, immune response and quality of life:

Link here:
https://pubmed.ncbi.nlm.nih.gov/36995535/

* * *

Study scope:

• Review of 39 clinical trials conducted between 2010 and 2020.

• Investigation of 12 different medicinal mushroom supplements in various types of cancer.

• Most commonly studied mushrooms: PSK (polysaccharide K) from the butterfly polypore (Trametes versicolor) (10 studies), shiitake mycelium extract (Lentinula edodes) (8 studies), Huaier granules (Trametes robiniophila Murr.) (5 studies), and AHCC (Active Hexose Correlated Compound, a proprietary shiitake extract) (5 studies).

• Other mushrooms studied: Reishi (Ganoderma lucidum), Maitake (Grifola frondosa), Phellinus linteus, Agaricus blazei, and Chaga (Inonotus obliquus).

• Most commonly studied cancers: stomach cancer (11 studies), breast cancer (8 studies), and prostate cancer (5 studies), with additionalstudies on colon, pancreatic, and esophageal cancer.

* * *

Survival Benefits:

• **Huaier Granules** improved overall survival (OS) and disease-free survival (DFS) in 2 hepatocellular carcinoma (HCC) studies and 1 breast cancer study.

• PSK, a beta-glucan from **butterfly mushroom**, improved survival outcomes in 4 gastric cancer studies when used as adjuvant therapy.

* * *

Immune System Modulation:

• 11 studies reported positive immune responses, including increased natural killer (NK) cell activity, T cell function, and cytokine regulation.

• These effects were particularly noted with PSK, Huaier Granules, and shiitake mycelium extract.

* * *

Improvements in quality of life (QoL):

• 14 studies found that mushroom supplementation resulted in a reduction in symptom burden, improved energy levels, and better overall well-being.

• Benefits were particularly evident in patients undergoing chemotherapy.

* * *

Adverse effects:

• Some studies reported mild side effects (grade 2 or lower), including nausea, vomiting, diarrhea, and muscle pain.

* * *

Study limitations:

• Many studies had small sample sizes and lacked randomized controlled trial (RCT) designs.

• Only one study was conducted in the United States, while most were conducted in Japan (20 studies), China (9 studies), Taiwan (2 studies), Brazil (2 studies), South Korea

(2 studies), and one each in Norway, Iraq, and Thailand.

• More large-scale, high-quality clinical trials are needed to confirm efficacy and safety for routine use in cancer treatment.

Mushrooms have tremendous potential for the prevention and treatment of cancer, both mechanistically, epidemiologically and clinically.

Large-scale, high-quality clinical trials should be initiated to further investigate the efficacy of mushrooms in cancer treatment.

In the meantime, including more mushrooms in your diet is a well-supported and proactive step that may help reduce cancer risk.

So far Nicolas Hulscher.

I disagree with his comments on limitations of the study.

- **Firstly**, there are actually thousands of studies on Huaier   and others, you just have to look for them.
- **Secondly**, many of them deal with the mechanisms of action, which in my view as a physicist makes more sense than huge studies that only look for correlations.

Hulscher is an epidemiologist and the big studies are the focus.

Anyone who can prove the mode of action has shown causality.

In this article, I reported on several studies that go into detail about the mechanisms of action.

Link to this:
https://tkp.at/2024/12/18/tcm-medikament-huaier-pilz-laut-studien-hochwirksam-gegen-krebs-und-impfschaeden/

Read the full report on page 62!

Read the full report on page 62!

* * *

The study by Tomasz Jędrzejewski et al

Source:
https://www.mdpi.com/1422-0067/24/5/4864

is titled "COVID-19 and Cancer Diseases—The Potential of Coriolus versicolor Mushroom to Combat Global Health Challenges."

A special focus of the study was placed on the mechanisms of direct action of Coriolus versicolo (CV) on cancer cells and angiogenesis.

A possible use of CV compounds in antiviral treatment, including therapy of COVID-19 disease, was also analyzed based on the latest literature.

The conclusions attest to the mushroom's very strong healing effects:
"This mushroom exhibits a wide range of benefits that can be useful in combating modern medical challenges.

We have presented data here that provide evidence of strong antiviral, anti-inflammatory, antioxidant and immune-stimulating properties of CV.
At the same time, other reports confirmed the impressive anti-cancer effect of CV extract and its compounds on a wide range of cancers and revealed the molecular background of this process.
By inducing various modalities of cell death, such as apoptosis or necroptosis, CV extract appears to be an effective adjuvant therapy.

In addition, analysis of other reports revealed that CV also affects fever, a mechanism of innate immunity that is beneficial for curing both cancer and viral infections."
So far this study.

Doctors experienced with medicinal mushrooms point out that a combination of medicinal mushrooms is useful: for example, the butterfly tramete with the chaga mushroom. In any case, one should not forget about supplementation of vitamins D and C, the consumption of which is high in practically any disease process.

* * *

COVID-19 and cancer diseases

The potential of the Coriolus versicolor mushroom to combat global health challenges Coriolus versicolor (CV) is a common species from the Polyporaceae family that has been used in traditional Chinese herbal medicine for over 2000 years. The most active compounds identified in CV include polysaccharide peptides such as

polysaccharide peptide (PSP) and polysaccharide-K (PSK, krestin), which are already used in some countries as adjuvant agents in cancer therapy.
This paper analyzes research progress in the field of the anticancer and antiviral effects of CV. The results of the data obtained in in vitro and in vivo studies using animal models as well as in clinical research studies were discussed.

The current update provides a brief overview of the immunomodulatory effects of CV.
A special focus is on the mechanisms of direct action of CV on cancer cells and angiogenesis.
A possible use of CV compounds in antiviral treatment, including therapy against COVID-19 disease, was also analyzed based on the latest literature.
In addition, the importance of fever in viral infections and cancer was discussed, suggesting that CV influences this phenomenon.

1. Introduction
Natural products have played an important role in healthcare since ancient times.
In academic medicine, there are many examples of drugs (including chemotherapeutics) derived from plants and fungi, e.g. B. Topotecan 1[1], etoposide, teniposide 2[2], docetaxel and paclitaxel [33].

Interestingly, the 2015 Nobel Prize for Medicine was awarded for artemisinin – the active ingredient of the medicinal herb "sweet wormwood" – which is an effective antimalarial therapy 4[4].
Read the complete article at the above source!!

TCM drug Huaier mushroom highly effective against cancer and vaccine damage according to studies

Source:
https://tkp.at/2024/12/18/tcm-medikament-huaier-pilz-laut-studien-hochwirksam-gegen-krebs-und-impfschaeden/
By Dr. Peter F. Mayer

One of the serious negative consequences of the corona vaccination campaign is cancer or turbo cancer.
This is evident from the databases in which vaccine damage is reported, as well as from studies and reports by oncologists.
The only known drug that is effective against vaccine damage and cancer is the Huaier mushroom, which has been used very successfully in traditional Chinese medicine for over 1000 years.

I became aware of the TCM drug Huaier mushroom through the study by **Tanaka et al** (2022).

In it, patients with stage 4 cancer were successfully treated with Huaier extract.

The mRNA vaccination came along and it was shown that Huaier can also prevent and even eliminate vaccine damage.
Patients who stopped taking Huaier after the vaccination experienced a new outbreak of cancer and died relatively quickly.

The patients who continued taking Huaier had no problems whatsoever.

The study's methodology consists of RNA sequencing. This shows which genes are active and what has changed as a result of the vaccination.
The most important finding is that the vaccination disrupts or even destroys the ribosomes and therefore various signaling pathways in the cell are massively weakened.

The destruction of the ribosomes is so crucially harmful because they are the protein factories of the cells.
For example, they produce enzymes - and without them there is no metabolism, the cell dies and then the body.
Florian Schilling explains this in detail in a recommended video, **which can be seen here in this article on the Huaier study.**

LINK:
https://tkp.at/2022/10/05/studie-c19-impfungen-fuehren-zu-vorzeitiger-zell-alterung-und-foerdern-krebserkrankung-video-mit-florian-schilling/
You can read the complete report on page 42.

* * *

A follow-up study (1) by Tanaka et al (2023) confirmed the results of the first and further clarified the mechanisms of action.

Source:
https://www.fortunejournals.com/articles/huaier-effects-on-prevention-and-inhibition-of-spontaneous-sarscov2-virion-production-by-repeated-pfizerbiontech-mrna-vaccination.html

TKP report here.
https://tkp.at/2023/05/30/japanische-studie-zeigt-wie-huaier-pilz-krebs-bekaempft-und-schaedliche-impf-spike-aus-dem-koerper-entfernt/
You can read the complete report on page 33.

Many studies confirm Huaier's high effectiveness
A search in the scientific publications brings up numerous hits from studies that confirm the effectiveness of Trametes Robiniophila Murr (Huaier) against various types of cancer.
For example, in the Journal of Ethnopharmacology dated November 15, 2024 by Hao Ji et al with the title
"The role and molecular mechanism of Trametes Robiniophila Murr(Huaier) in tumor therapy"

Source:
https://pmc.ncbi.nlm.nih.gov/articles/PMC7737552/

The role and molecular mechanism of Trametes Robiniophila Murr (Huaier) in tumor therapy).
The study provides an overview of current research results including findings on the mechanisms of action.
It states that Trametes Robiniophila Murr has been extensively documented in ethnopharmacological research in China.

Huaier has been used clinically in China for over 1000 years.
Traditional clinical application reports demonstrate the widespread use of Huaier to treat various types of cancer and to strengthen the autoimmunity of tumor patients.

Trametes Robiniophila Murr (Huaier), a traditional Chinese medicine, has been shown to be extremely effective in the clinical treatment of various tumors.

The main bioactive components of Huaier are mushroom-like compounds, including polysaccharides, proteins, ketones, alkaloids and minerals.

The research results show that Huaier serves as a reliable therapeutic tool by effectively inhibiting the proliferation of cancer cells, inducing apoptosis in cancer cells, suppressing tumor metastasis, regulating tumor stem cells and controlling immune function.

Therefore, it exerts a strong antitumor effect when used in conjunction with conventional cancer therapies.
A December 2020 study also provides an overview of the mechanisms of action.

Under the title **"Research Progress on the Anti-Cancer Molecular Mechanisms of Huaier"**, Tongton Qi et al explain the mechanisms of action in breast cancer, gastrointestinal cancer, liver cancer, and lung cancer.

Link:
https://www.spandidos-publications.com/10.3892/or.2015.3950

In kidney cancer and some other types of cancer.

"Microarray gene analysis shows that Huaier has multiple targets to achieve anti-tumor effects, including curbing proliferation and metastasis, disrupting cell cycle, inducing apoptosis, pyrose and autophagy, inhibiting intratumoral angiogenesis, attenuating tumor stem cell-like cell properties, impairing tumor-related immune system function, reversing drug resistance and increasing sensitivity to other chemotherapeutic agents, etc.
More broadly, Huaier exhibits these biological effects by regulating specific pathway-related proteins targeting oncogenes and tumor suppressor genes and/or by influencing gene expression through ncRNA."

The anti-cancer effect of Huaier mushrooms was shown, for example, **in this study from 2015 or in this study from August 2020** entitled "**Trametes robiniophila Murr in the treatment of breast cancer**" -
the scientific name of the Huaier mushroom is used here.

The graphic abstract of the article shows the findings on the mode of action.

Link to this:
https://www.sciencedirect.com/science/article/abs/pii/S0378874124008778

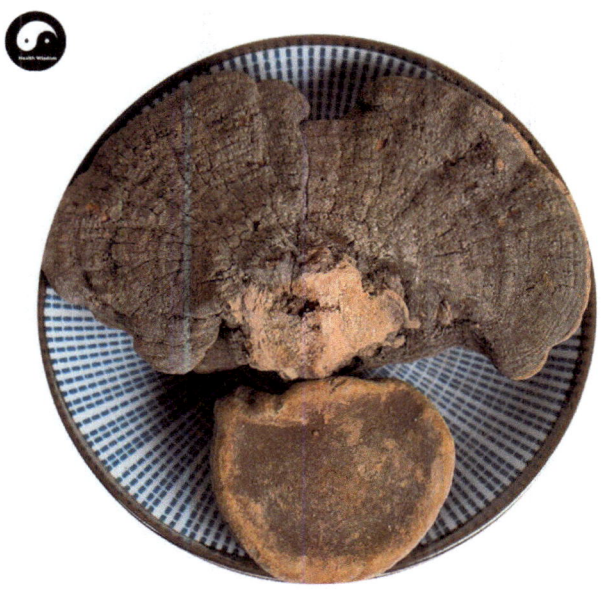

* * *

Here is another section from the abstract of the study:

"This systematic review focuses on the treatment of breast cancer and summarizes the healing effects of aqueous Huaier extract and polysaccharides in preclinical studies.
Huaier can significantly inhibit the progression of breast cancer with low toxicity, improve the immune response and increase sensitivity to radiation and chemotherapy.
The therapeutic effect of Huaier granules in clinical studies was also taken into account.

67

This review summarizes the current studies and highlights the promising role of Huaier and its polysaccharides as a complementary alternative medicine in breast cancer treatment."

* * *

According to reports from doctors, the strigiliform tramete, which is also native to Europe, has a similar effect.

In studies, an alcoholic and aqueous extract is almost always used.
As a powder in tea or other drinks, it hardly changes the taste.

* * *

Here is a small excerpt from the large number of other studies from the very active research scene:

Molecular mechanisms and therapeutic applications of Huaier in cancer treatment Jan 12, 2024 Huaier improves the efficacy of anti-PD-L1 Ab in the treatment of hepatocellular carcinoma by regulating the immunological microenvironment of the tumor Jan 1, 2024 Immunoregulatory effects of Huaier (Trametes robiniophila Murr) and relevant clinical applications June 28, 2023

Medicinal mushroom supplements in cancer:

A systematic review of clinical trials March 30, 2023
The potential therapeutic benefits of Huaier in digestive
system cancer: Its chemical constituents,
pharmacological applications and future direction July 1,
2024
Huaier partially inhibits the proliferative and invasive
potential of human hepatoma SKHEP-1 cells due to
reduced Lamin B1 and increased NOV August 9, 2016

* * *

Study from Japan: Strong evidence of a connection between cancer and mRNA

Link to this:
https://tkp.at/2025/02/12/studie-aus-japan-starker-beleg-fuer-zusammenhang-von-krebs-und-mrna/
Author: Dr. Peter F. Mayer

In 2022 and 2023, more people died of cancer in Japan than usual.
This is the result of a recently published paper and suggests a connection to the mRNA vaccination.

In Japan, there were around 12,000 more cancer deaths in 2022 and 2023 than expected, Japanese researchers reported in a preprint this week.
That is two percent more deaths than expected, which means statistical significance and rather rules out coincidence.
The study is the strongest evidence yet that mRNA vaccines can cause cancer in some people.

Link to this:
https://zenodo.org/records/14847943

The cancer that caused the most additional deaths was leukemia.
A type of cancer that relates directly to the immune system and may be most directly affected by the mRNAs.
Leukemia deaths increased by 8 percent annually, totaling over 1,300 additional deaths.
On a monthly basis, the sequence is striking, with

leukemia deaths increasing significantly after vaccinations began in 2021.

The researchers acknowledged that they cannot prove that mRNA vaccines caused the increase in deaths. But they called for an "urgent" investigation.

* * *

US journalist Alex Berenson is currently reporting on the paper:

Link to this:

https://alexberenson.substack.com/p/urgent-cancer-deaths-rose-in-japan?utm_source=post-email-title&publication_id=363080&post_id=156929538&utm_campaign=email-post-title&isFreemail=true&r=18rnaa&triedRedirect=true&utm_medium=email

The figures from Japan are particularly important because Japan used almost exclusively mRNA-based Covid vaccines and had a high vaccination rate.

In addition, the country has an excellent medical system and a relatively healthy population, so there are fewer confounding factors - known or unknown variables that could distort these results.

The likelihood of dying from cancer increases with age, and Japan's population is aging rapidly.
Therefore, demographic researchers must take into account the average age of the population to fairly compare year-to-year changes.

The researchers did this, using similar procedures to official Japanese government agencies.

They reported 7,160 additional deaths in 2022 - about 2.1 percent above the expected total – and 4,730 in 2023, 1.4 percent above expectations.

* * *

(mRNA vaccinations), then leukemia.

The chart on the right shows the annual leukemia death rates in Japan, adjusted for age.
The chart on the left shows the monthly deviations from the norm - in the red bars - plotted against Japan's vaccination cycles, the lower blue graph)

You can see the graph on the next page of the book!

In addition to **leukemia**, there were also statistically significant increases in several other cancers, including **prostate** and **oral cancer.**
Skin cancer increased significantly in 2023, but the increase did not quite reach statistical significance.

Deaths from ovarian cancer increased even more than those from leukemia compared to baseline, but ovarian cancer is less common than leukemia, so the absolute increase was smaller, at about 900 additional deaths.

The researchers acknowledged that they did not know the vaccination status of those who died and therefore could not directly link the increase in deaths to the mRNAs.

However, given the predictability of cancer deaths and the frequency of Covid vaccinations in Japan in 2021 and 2022, it is statistically very unlikely that even a small increase could have occurred if vaccinated people had not made up the vast majority of those affected.

In their discussion, the researchers pointed to several possible biological pathways by which the mRNAs could cause cancer.

Although none of these are proven, the increase in cancer deaths - which has now continued for two years in one of the world's largest industrialized countries - can no longer be ignored, they write.

"The timing requires urgent and rigorous investigations, including analyzes by vaccination status and clinical validation," they write.

(B) leukemia : annual and monthly

German cancer researchers: Vitamin D protects against cancer - and also against Covid

Link to this:
https://tkp.at/2021/02/13/deutsche-krebsforscher-vitamin-d-schuetzt-vor-krebs-und-uebrigens-auch-vor-covid/
Author: Dr. Peter F Mayer

The 2018 Nobel Prize in Medicine was awarded for research that showed how cancer can be fought by strengthening the immune system.
The German vitamin D "pope", Prof. Jörg Spitz (videos below), has been pointing out for years that vitamin D prevents and fights cancer - provided you have a sufficiently high level.
Spitz also points out that vitamin D is the most important preventive measure to prevent infection with the coronavirus and more serious illnesses.

The renowned German Cancer Research Center (DKFZ) is now also showing the benefits in cancer treatment and prevention. Since it is funded 90% by the Federal Ministry of Education and Research and 10% by the state of Baden-Württemberg, it can apparently operate independently of third-party funding and is therefore not subject to the interests of the pharmaceutical industry.

A press release states that three meta-analyses of clinical studies in recent years have concluded that vitamin D supplementation is associated with a reduction in the death rate from cancer by around 13 percent.

Link to this:

https://www.dkfz.de/aktuelles/pressemitigungen/detail/
vitamin-d-supplementierung-moeglicher-gewinn-an-
lebensjahren-bei-gleichzeitiger-kostenersparnis

Scientists at the DKFZ have now applied these results to the situation in Germany and calculated that if all Germans over 50 years of age were given vitamin D supplementation, up to 30,000 cancer deaths per year could potentially be avoided and more than 300,000 years of life could be gained – while at the same time saving costs.

* * *

Vitamin D protects against a number of diseases

For several years, scientists have been studying the influence of an adequate vitamin D supply on the prognosis of numerous diseases.
The focus is particularly on inflammatory diseases, diabetes, respiratory diseases and cancer, according to the DKFZ.

The studies on cancer mortality came to a consistent conclusion: vitamin D supplementation reduces cancer mortality by around 13 percent - across all types of cancer.
The biological mechanisms underlying this have not yet been clarified.
Only methodologically high-quality randomized studies from all parts of the world were included in the meta-analyses.

"In many countries around the world, age-adjusted cancer mortality has fortunately fallen in the last decade," says Hermann Brenner, epidemiologist at the German Cancer Research Center (DKFZ).

"However, given the often considerable costs of many new cancer drugs, this success often comes at a high price.
Vitamin D, on the other hand, is comparatively inexpensive in the usual daily doses."

* * *

Vitamin D supplementation saves costs

Vitamin D deficiency is widespread among older people and especially among cancer patients. Brenner and colleagues now calculated the costs that would arise from vitamin D supplementation for the entire population of Germany over the age of 50.
They compared this sum with the possible savings in cancer treatments, which often cost tens of thousands of euros, especially in the case of advanced cancer in the last months of the patient's life.

For this calculation, the scientists assumed a daily dose of 1000 international units of vitamin D at a price of 25 euros per person per year.
In 2016, there were around 36 million people over the age of 50 living in Germany, which results in annual costs for supplementation of 900 million euros.

(**Note**: I use 10,000 IU daily in winter, and considerably less in summer - the cost: 25 euros per year.)
Dr. Peter F. Mayer

The researchers took the costs of cancer treatment from the scientific literature and assumed average additional treatment costs of €40,000 for the last year of life of the patients who died of cancer alone.
A 13 percent reduction in cancer mortality in Germany corresponded to around 30,000 fewer cancer-related deaths per year, the treatment costs of which amounted to €1.154 billion in the model calculation.

Compared to the costs of vitamin supplementation, this model calculates annual savings of €254 million.
Vitamin D supplementation used successfully in countries such as Finland.

The researchers determined the number of years of life lost at the time of cancer death using the mortality tables of the Federal Statistical Office.
Brenner believes that the cost and effort of routinely determining vitamin D levels are unnecessary, as there is no risk of overdose with a supplement of 1000 international units.
Such a prior determination was not carried out in the clinical studies either.

Brenner summarizes:

> "In view of the potentially significant positive effects on cancer mortality - coupled with possible cost savings - we should look for new

ways to reduce the vitamin D deficiency that is widespread in the elderly population in Germany. In some countries, food has even been fortified with vitamin D for many years - for example in Finland, where cancer death rates are around 20 percent lower than in Germany.

Not to mention that there is increasing evidence of other positive health effects of an adequate vitamin D supply, for example in the death rates from lung diseases. Finally, we believe that vitamin D supplementation is so safe that we even recommend it for newborn babies to develop healthy bones."

It should also be added about Finland that it is one of the countries with the fewest Covid deaths in Europe - less than a tenth of the European average.
Finland is roughly on a par with countries such as Belarus (with measures similar to Sweden), Norway, Iceland and India.

The German Cancer Research Center (DKFZ) is the largest biomedical research facility in Germany with more than 3,000 employees.
Over 1,300 scientists at the DKFZ are researching how cancer develops, recording cancer risk factors and looking for new strategies to prevent people from developing cancer.
They are developing new methods with which tumors can be diagnosed more precisely and cancer patients treated more successfully.

And here are the videos both directly about vitamin D and corona as well as another one below from a somewhat broader lecture given on February 27, 2018 in Vienna:

Links to this:
https://www.youtube.com/watch?v=JcZ2_8htKSw

https://www.youtube.com/watch?v=xEU7Hb8KrpM

* * *

Masks could promote the growth of cancer

Link to this:
https://tkp.at/2022/06/17/masken-koennten-das-wachstum-von-krebs-foerdern/
Author: Dr. Peter F. Mayer

It is no longer news that the "experts" have lied to the public about masks. It has been proven time and time again that masks and the constraints imposed by frightened politicians do not work.
And yet the untruths spread by the "experts" and their allies in the media have become permanently entrenched in a large part of the population.
But there could well be other unrecognized dangers associated with them.

I would like to link two facts to this. First of all, it is about the change in the CO2 content in the air we breathe due to masks.
Masks increase the dead space from which the exhaled air with a high CO2 content is rebreathed.
The average dead space volume during breathing is around 150-180 mL in adults and is significantly increased when wearing a mask that covers the mouth and nose. For example, an experimental study using an FFP2/N95 mask found the dead space volume to be around 98-168 mL.

This corresponds to a mask-related increase in dead space of around 65 to 112% in adults and thus almost a doubling.

The air at the Sonnblick Observatory at an altitude of 3000 meters contains around 420 ppm (parts per million) (0.042%) oxygen. The exhaled air contains a fairly constant around 4% or 40,000 ppm CO_2.
Room air usually has around 460 to 470 ppm, although this depends heavily on the ventilation and the number of CO_2 producers in the room.

I know of more than 10 studies in which the CO_2 concentration in the air breathed was measured behind masks. The following values were fairly consistent:

Art	Erwachsene	Kinder
Chirurgische Maske	5.000 ppm	6.500 ppm
FFP2 / N95	9.500 ppm	13.000 ppm

One of the studies was retracted after unscientific criticism by Jama Pediatrics, but without providing measurements that would prove other values.

Link to this:
https://jamanetwork.com/journals/jamapediatrics/fullarticle/2781743
Text in English!

This is the usual procedure in natural science, but of course not in medicine, which is controlled by pharmaceutical interests. One has not yet been peer-reviewed and a further 11 studies are summarized in this meta-study.

Links to this:
https://www.medrxiv.org/content/
10.1101/2022.05.10.22274813v1

https://www.mdpi.com/1660-4601/18/8/4344
Text in English!

A similar result was found for the drop in oxygen saturation and the impairment of breathing in six of the studies evaluated in this work.

* * *

Some interesting facts about cancer

We have known for about 100 years that tumor cells feed by fermenting sugar, i.e. without oxygen.
This finding comes from the German biochemist Professor Otto Warburg (Nobel Prize 1931).
Warburg was able to show that the cancer cell lives primarily on sugar and - although there is enough oxygen - ferments it without oxygen.

Oxygen present – fermentation without oxygen.
With a rather poor energy yield.
At the University of Graz, Professor Frank Madeo was able to show that:

      • the reduction of cell respiration (i.e.
      shortness of breath) reduces the programmed,

natural cell death, known as apoptosis, and therefore allows cells to live uncontrollably.

• Uncontrolled survival means rapid growth, which means cancer.

Prof. Madeo:
"This increased resistance (to cell death) could contribute significantly to tumor formation and malignancy (metastasis)."

The study entitled "The Warburg Effect Suppresses Oxidative Stress Induced Apoptosis in a Yeast Model for Cancer" was published in Plos One.

Link to this:
https://journals.plos.org/plosone/article?id=10.1371/journal.pone.0004592

With this model, the Graz researchers were able to prove that cells have a survival advantage due to the so-called Warburg effect.
So
• aggressive cancer cells feed on sugar (glycolysis)

• while simultaneously reducing oxygen respiration.

Increased respiratory activity, i.e. more oxygen supply, inhibits the growth of tumors. According to Madeo.

The slim university professor goes on to explain:

"Interestingly, endurance sports are one of the best preventive measures against cancer.
This increases the body's oxygen supply and also consumes sugar.
Both, according to the classic Warburg hypothesis, are poison for the cancer cell."

The conclusion of the study is:
"The Warburg effect could therefore contribute directly to the development of cancer - not only through increased glycolysis, but also through reduced respiration in the presence of oxygen, which suppresses apoptosis."

However, compulsory mask wearing reduces the oxygen content and increases that of carbon dioxide.
This is exactly the opposite of what protects against cancer.

The number of cancer cases has increased significantly since autumn 2020, or at least since the start of the vaccination campaign.
The masks could be one of the reasons for this.

Mushrooms work against dementia and strengthen the immune system

Link to this:
https://tkp.at/2024/04/04/pilze-wirken-gegen-demenz-und-staerken-das-immunsystem/
Author: Dr. Peter F. Mayer

In 2022, studies had shown that mushrooms are effective anti-cancer agents and can even prevent the negative consequences of vaccination spikes. The two Japanese studies used Huaier (Trametes robiniophila murr), which is available in China but not here.

But a number of other mushrooms also have strong health effects, prevent diseases, strengthen and regulate the immune system.

I reported on the second Japanese study here, on the first in this article including the explanatory video by Florian Schilling.
Studies had already shown the effectiveness of mushrooms earlier.
This study by researchers at the National University of Singapore (NUS) found that older adults who consume more mushrooms in their diet have a significantly lower risk of mild cognitive impairment than those who do not (title: "Eating mushrooms may reduce the risk of cognitive decline")

Links to this:
https://tkp.at/2023/05/30/japanische-studie-zeigt-wie-huaier-pilz-krebs-bekaempft-und-schaedliche-impf-spike-aus-dem-koerper-entfernt/
Read the full report on page 33!

https://tkp.at/2022/10/05/studie-c19-impfungen-fuehren-zu-vorzeitiger-zell-alterung-und-foerdern-krebserkrankung-video-mit-florian-schilling/
Read the full report on page 42!

https://www.sciencedaily.com/releases/2019/03/190312103702.htm

Mild cognitive impairment is a condition defined by experts as the stage between the expected cognitive decline that occurs with age and the more serious decline caused by dementia.

Link to this:
https://www.mayoclinic.org/diseases-conditions/mild-cognitive-impairment/symptoms-causes/syc-20354578

Although mild cognitive impairment can increase an adult's risk of developing Alzheimer's, the condition can be prevented or treated with healthy lifestyle and dietary changes.

Research suggests there is no single cause for mild cognitive impairment, but certain changes in the structure of the brain are commonly seen in people with the condition.

The same changes are also seen in the brains of people with Alzheimer's or other forms of dementia, although to a lesser extent. Diabetes, stroke, or depression increase the likelihood that a person will develop mild cognitive impairment.

Link to this:
https://www.nia.nih.gov/health/memory-loss-and-forgetfulness/what-mild-cognitive-impairment

Although the symptoms of mild cognitive impairment are not as severe as those of Alzheimer's or dementia, the condition can still affect quality of life.
Common signs of mild cognitive impairment include forgetfulness, difficulty finding words, and frequently losing things.
However, unlike people with Alzheimer's, people with mild cognitive impairment do not experience personality changes and can still carry out their daily activities independently.

* * *

A diet rich in mushrooms may help prevent mild cognitive impairment.

To understand how eating mushrooms may affect brain function, NUS researchers analyzed data from 663 Singaporeans aged 60 and above.
The six-year study, published in the Journal of Alzheimer's Disease, was conducted from 2011 to 2017 and specifically looked at the amount of mushrooms participants consumed per week.

(**Title**: The Association between Mushroom Consumption and Mild Cognitive Impairment: A Community-Based Cross-Sectional Study in Singapore)

Link here:
https://content.iospress.com/articles/journal-of-alzheimers-disease/jad180959

The researchers found that compared to participants who ate mushrooms less than once a week, those who consumed more than two servings of mushrooms per week had a 50 percent lower risk of mild cognitive impairment.
This association was independent of age, gender, education, alcohol consumption, smoking habits, physical and social activities, and other conditions such as high blood pressure, stroke, diabetes, and heart disease.

For comparison, one serving is 3/4 cup of cooked mushrooms, weighing about 150 grams (g).
Two servings are about half a plate of cooked mushrooms.
That's how much you should eat in a week to reduce the likelihood of mild cognitive impairment, according to the study.
Eating just a small portion of mushrooms per week can go a long way toward maintaining brain health.

Mushrooms are a versatile and nutritious culinary ingredient because they are one of the few dietary sources of **ergosterol**.
This compound is converted to vitamin D2 when exposed to ultraviolet (UV) light.

A cup of mushrooms can also provide many other nutrients, such as protein, copper, B vitamins, potassium and iron.

I have the PDF file for ergosterol. I can send it to you if you wish.
Please write to me at: traude-schubert@gmx.de

Link to ... many other nutrients provide...
https://www.verywellfit.com/mushroom-nutrition-facts-calories-and-health-benefits-4117115

Most importantly, the NUS researchers believe that the brain-boosting effects of mushrooms are due to ergothioneine, an amino acid found in almost all types of mushrooms.

"Ergothioneine is a unique antioxidant and anti-inflammatory that humans cannot synthesize. However, it can be obtained from food, especially mushrooms," explained Dr. Irwin Cheah, one of the study's authors.

According to a recent study published in the journal FEBS Letters, ergothioneine has shown antidepressant effects in mice and memory-enhancing effects in humans.

Related links:
https://beatdepression.news/

https://febs.onlinelibrary.wiley.com/doi/10.1002/1873-3468.14271

The beneficial effects on the brain can be attributed to its ability to protect brain cells (neurons) from oxidative damage and promote neurogenesis (formation of new neurons) and neuronal maturation.

Other bioactive compounds in mushrooms, such as hericenone, erinacine, scabronine and dictyophorine, may also promote the synthesis of neuronal growth factors and reduce the risk of cognitive decline.

* * *

6 Mushrooms That Support the Brain

There are about 200 known edible mushrooms. To improve brain health, include these six of the best mushrooms that science says support healthy brain function in your diet.

Chaga mushroom (Inonotus obliquus)

According to a study published in the International Journal of Biological Macromolecules, the Chaga mushroom contains a bioactive polysaccharide that can protect against Alzheimer's disease by increasing the expression of Nrf2 in the brain.
Nrf2 is a protein that is "responsible for regulating a variety of antioxidant enzymes" that are involved in detoxification and combating oxidative stress. Basically,

Chaga therefore has a regulating effect on the immune system.

Link to this:
https://www.sciencedirect.com/science/article/abs/pii/S0141813019304672

https://www.mdpi.com/2076-3921/10/9/1479

The susceptibility of the brain to oxidative stress is a key damaging factor in Alzheimer's disease.

Link to this:
https://www.mdpi.com/2076-3921/10/9/1479

Chaga has been known as an anti-cancer agent for centuries in northern countries, where the most effective products come from.
Chaga mushrooms are fungi that grow on the bark of various trees, such as birch (pictured above).
These mushrooms are commonly found in countries such as Siberia, Russia, Korea and Canada.

Chaga mushrooms are often overlooked because they look like random pieces of charcoal hanging from a tree.
Chaga mushrooms are used in cancer therapies to slow the growth of cancer cells.

Test-tube studies have shown that chaga extract can inhibit the growth of liver, lung, breast, prostate and colon cancer cells.

Link to this:
https://naturalpedia.com/colon-cancer-causes-side-effects-and-treatments-at-naturalpedia-com.html

In addition, animal studies show that supplementing with chaga can reduce tumor size by up to 60 percent.
Chaga mushrooms contain antioxidants that can protect cells from free radical damage.
The antioxidant triterpene in particular is known to have the ability to kill cancer cells. Research has shown that Chaga extract can regulate the production of special proteins called cytokines.
These proteins play a role in stimulating white blood cells, which protect the body from harmful pathogens such as bacteria and viruses - again, the function of regulating the immune system!

* * *

Oyster mushroom (Pleurotus ostreatus)

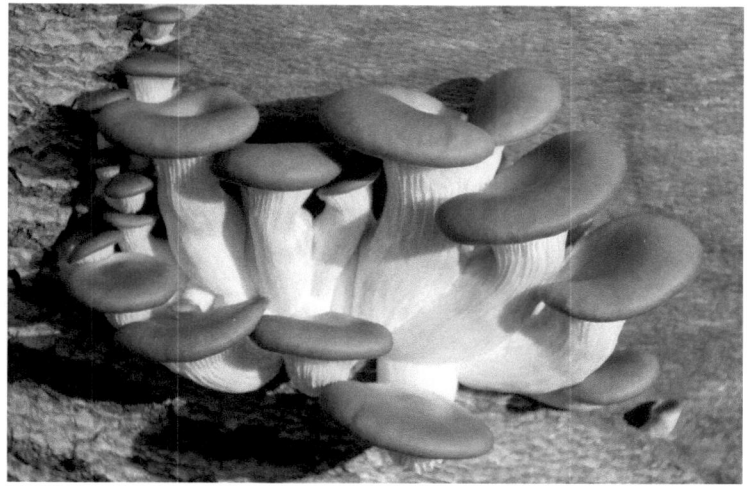

In traditional Chinese medicine (TCM), oyster mushroom is often used to relax muscles, tendons and joints. Research has shown that oyster mushroom, like Chaga, can help reduce oxidative stress in the brain.

Link to this:
https://www.sciencedirect.com/science/article/abs/pii/S0009279708004018?via%3Dihub

According to a study by Indian researchers, oyster mushrooms contain compounds that can protect against oxidative damage by increasing the levels of antioxidants such as vitamin C and glutathione, as well as various antioxidant enzymes in the brain in response to stress factors.

* * *

Lion's Mane (Hericium erinaceus)

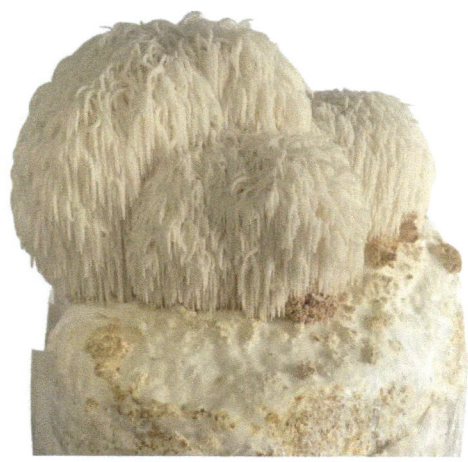

When it comes to supporting a healthy brain and nervous system, lion's mane is considered one of the best mushrooms to eat.

Studies show that the hericenones and erinacines contained in lion's mane can stimulate the expression of nerve growth factors, which help regulate the growth, development and maintenance of neurons in the brain.

Link to this:
https://onlinelibrary.wiley.com/doi/10.1155/2018/5802634

A clinical study involving Japanese adults with mild cognitive impairment also found that other components of lion's mane, particularly in its fruiting body where the hericenones are concentrated, may contribute to its neuroprotective benefits.

Maitake (Grifola frondosa)

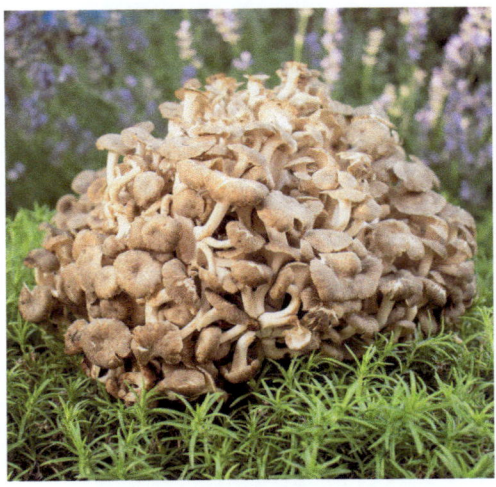

Maitake is widely considered a superfood due to its richness in important nutrients.

Link to this:
https://www.mdpi.com/2304-8158/10/1/95

These include:
-        proteins,
-        fiber,
-        carbohydrates,
-        the vitamin D2 precursor ergosterol
-        and minerals such as
-        potassium,
-        phosphorus,
-        calcium
-        and magnesium.

According to a study published in the journal RSC

Advances, maitake contains a polysaccharide called proteo-B-glucan, which has powerful immunomodulatory and neuroprotective properties.

Link to this:
https://pubs.rsc.org/en/content/articlelanding/2019/ra/c9ra08245j
The report is in English!

Proteo-B-glucan was found to improve Alzheimer's disease-like pathology, as well as memory and learning impairments, by promoting the breakdown of amyloid-B plaques in the brain.

* * *

Reishi (Ganoderma lucidum)

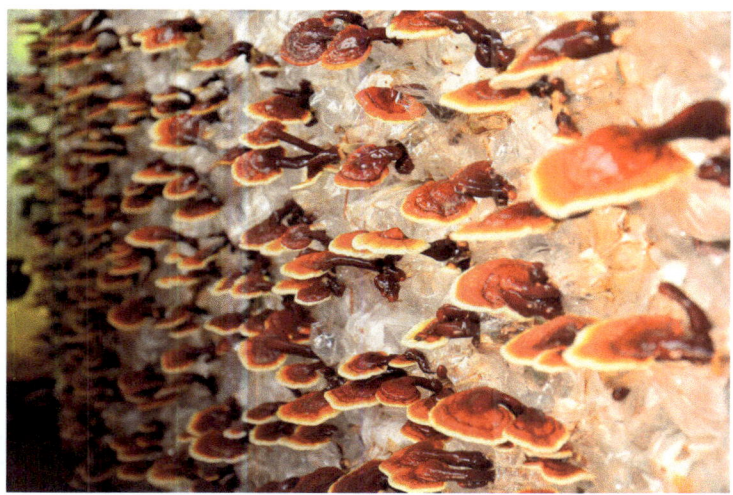

Reishi, also known by its Chinese name Lingzhi, is a medicinal mushroom known for its numerous health benefits, including boosting the immune system, fighting cancer, reducing fatigue and depression, and supporting optimal brain function.

Link to this:
https://www.healthline.com/nutrition/reishi-mushroom-benefits

According to a study published in Frontiers in Aging Neuroscience, the reishi mushroom contains powerful triterpenoids that can mitigate age-related physiological brain decline.
Specifically, the compound ganoderic acid A was found to improve brain function in mice with Alzheimer's disease

because it promotes the elimination of pathological metabolic products that can damage the brain.

Link to this:
https://www.frontiersin.org/journals/aging-neuroscience/articles/10.3389/fnagi.2021.628860/full

* * *

Shiitake (Lentinula edodes)

A study conducted by Chinese researchers found that consuming shiitake may help prevent cognitive impairment caused by a high-fat diet.

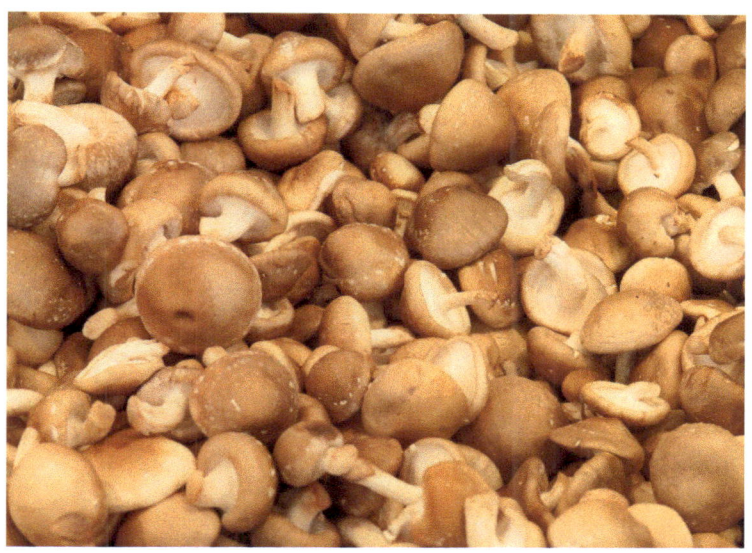

Link to this:
https://translational-medicine.biomedcentral.com/
articles/10.1186/s12967-021-02724-6

It is said that a high-fat diet over time leads to changes in the gut microbiota that can trigger inflammation in the brain.
However, the study found that the beta-glucan in shiitake can prevent this harmful change in the composition of the gut microbiome, thus protecting the brain from damage that leads to impaired cognitive functions.
Mushrooms are nutritious and versatile ingredients that can easily be incorporated into various recipes. And I think they taste very good too.
The film "Fantastic Mushrooms - The Magical World at Our Feet" offers an exciting insight into the world of mushrooms.

Link to this:

https://www.amazon.de/Fantastic-Pilze-magische-unseren-F%C3%BC%C3%9Fen/dp/B09K1T5YCW?__mk_de_ DE=%C3%85M%C3%85%C5%BD%C3%95%C3%91&crid=BV7CXWHMMIRV&dib=eyJ2Ijoi MSJ9.5l9pIfRLDRrzW1NmSe8H62E3yIuKJX4Yim3nQG4 hzAkhP-qVGIAjE1DufV0cz1gPME_qhQ7Ocl8FKw5Z UeyIZd6jkWAL1VU3Wby4-cMa_i5qsnXvyT1_vZOK3c VPouz4PauhKFdPoWK23QqCBGHGrmcyd3l9uwaOi6ke WsjOn2ZNt9Qtk8m6A-Z9JyI4EKHjNKPbJmFwG V6RuO4a4wIUMmgiqGN 2yo6RaJgblN98ZR8. W2puAOv6hH-gj4UnW-nPbt8N77BQoCFzQacHL 3om42E&dib_tag=se&keywords=Fantastic+mushrooms+-+The+magical+world+at+our+feet&qid=1712212452 &sbo=RZvfv//HxDF%2BO5021pAnSA%3D %3D&sprefix=fantastic+mushrooms+-the+magical+world +at+our+feet,aps,205&sr=8-2&linkCode=sl1&tag=tkpat-21&linkId=2b18828cd05204019ac8c49191fc8a24&language=de_DE&ref_=as_li_ss_tl

Restrictions on the use of natural products for healing and health care

Link to this report:
https://tkp.at/2023/07/15/einschraenkungen-der-verwendung-von-naturprodukten-fuer-heilung-und-gesundheitsvorsorge/
Author: Dr. Peter F. Mayer

The pharmaceutical industry and its lobbyists in the authorities and medical institutions are waging a battle against effective natural products, dietary supplements, vitamins, homeopathy and everything that is useful but cannot be patented and therefore reduces profits.
Natural products are usually far more effective than drugs derived from them and without the side effects associated with pharmaceutical products.
Health Canada is now in the process of restricting the use of natural products.

The Natural Health Products Protection Association in Canada is mobilizing against a new pharmaceutical promotion project by the Canadian health authority.

Link to this:
https://nhppa.org/

They report on the next steps under Health Canada's Self-Care Framework, which are:

- restricting the use of natural products;

• removing the right to invoke traditional use of products to obtain approval to sell them, and

• fully applying the chemical drug regulations to natural health products.

These three changes will completely destroy the availability of natural health products. Most of the effective products will disappear.
Naturopathic practitioners such as naturopathic doctors, traditional Chinese doctors, homeopathic doctors, herbalists, nutritionists, etc. will lose their livelihoods.

These practitioners will have to go out of business because they will lose the natural remedies they use to help us.

Health Canada is imposing new fees on naturopathic companies that will put many small and medium-sized companies out of business.
Their products will disappear.

For those products that survive, prices will rise because manufacturers will have to pass on their increased costs. This will take the remaining products away from the poor and disadvantaged who cannot afford the higher prices.

The new fees Health Canada is charging will be used to create a new enforcement body to enforce the stricter regulations and censor truthful health information.

Manufacturers and practitioners will no longer be able to publicly disseminate truthful information about natural products.

Huge new fines will be imposed to cripple and destroy the natural health community.
Fines of $5,000,000 per day that Health Canada said were only appropriate for big pharmaceutical companies have now been imposed on natural health as well.

> - A local natural health store cannot survive a $5,000,000 fine.

> - A natural health practitioner, e.g. a naturopathic doctor, cannot survive a fine of $5,000,000.

These high fines are not intended to punish, but to destroy.

* * *

Restrictions in the EU

There are already restrictions in the EU too and attempts to expand them.

One example is the Huaier mushroom (Trametes robiniophila Murr).
Studies have shown that it is highly effective against cancer and against vaccine damage, because it reliably

removes the spike proteins that remain in the body as a result of multiple vaccinations.

TKP has reported on this in detail here:
Japanese study shows how Huaier mushroom fights cancer and removes harmful vaccination spikes from the body

Link to this:
https://tkp.at/2023/05/30/japanische-studie-zeigt-wie-huaier-pilz-krebs-bekaempft-und-schaedliche-impf-spike-aus-dem-koerper-entfernt/
You can read the full report on page 33!

https://tkp.at/2022/10/05/studie-c19-impfungen-fuehren-zu-vorzeitiger-zell-alterung-und-foerdern-krebserkrankung-video-mit-florian-schilling/
You can read the full report on page 42.

* * *

The Huaier mushroom, unlike the other tramete species, is only found in China and Japan and it is also quite rare. In China, however, it has been successfully cultivated and is certified as a medicine, but in Japan it is simply a food supplement.
The Huaier mushroom is not permitted in the EU on the basis of legal regulations, nor is the strigid tramete, which can be found in our forests and has similar effects to the Huaier.

Link to this:
https://www.efsa.europa.eu/de/topics/topic/novel-food

This is not a question of whether it is native or not, but rather of politicians arbitrarily allowing or banning certain foods.

As is usual in the EU, this depends largely on whether the respective producer can afford to send lobbyists to Brussels at great expense, who then influence politics in one direction or the other.

The full text of the law can be found on the European Commission website.

Link to this:

https://eur-lex.europa.eu/legal-content/DE/TXT/?uri=CELEX:32015R2283

However, Trametes versicolor (butterfly bracket fungus) or Chaga (Inonotus obliquus, also known as slate fungus) are permitted and available in the EU and are said to have similarly good effects against cancer and other ailments.

Links to this:

https://www.amazon.de/s?k=schmetterlingstramete&language=de_DE&crid=MCAF5RS11XU&linkCode=sl2&linkId=ba0b30f651e49e4e5a128f1eaf0399f1&sprefix=schmetterlingstramet%2Caps%2C107&tag=tkpat-21&ref=as_li_ss_tl

https://www.amazon.de/s?k=chaga+pilz&language=de_DE&crid=XAO2F82YLQGP&linkCode=sl2&linkId=9f3d30e2dc62232f87f504952cb67703&sprefix=chaga%2Caps%2C118&tag=tkpat-21&ref=as_li_ss_tl

Ultimately all this amounts to a restriction of patients' free choice regarding their treatment.

Note from me:
This must not happen under any circumstances.
Everyone has the right to decide for themselves!

Image sources

Cover
https://www.piqsels.com/de/public-domain-photo-fydpv

Reishi mushrooms
https://www.piqsels.com/de/public-domain-photo-srkfv/

Shiitake
https://www.piqsels.com/de/public-domain-photo-fjwyf

Oyster mushrooms
https://www.piqsels.com/de/public-domain-photo-otymd

Lion's mane + Maitake

Mushroom cultivation

Anti-cancer potential
https://tkp.at/2024/05/08/schmetterlings-tramete-hilft-gegen-krebs-studien/

Huaeir mushroom
https://tkp.at/2024/12/18/tcm-medikament-huaier-pilz-laut-studien-hochwirksam-gegen-krebs-und-impfschaeden/

Leukemia
https://tkp.at/2025/02/12/studie-aus-japan-starker-beleg-fuer-zusammenhang-von-krebs-und-mrna/

The molecular characterization ..
https://tkp.at/2023/05/30/japanische-studie-zeigt-wie-huaier-pilz-krebs-bekaempft-und-schaedliche-impf-spike-aus-dem-koerper-entfernt/

Book Mushrooms
https://www.amazon.de/Fantastische-Pilze-magische-unseren-F%C3%BC%C3%9Fen/dp/B09K1T5YCW?__mk_de_DE=%C3%85M%C3%85%C5%BD%C3%95%C3%91&crid=BV7CXWHMMIRV&dib=eyJ2Ijoi
MSJ9.5l9pIfRLDRrzW1NmSe8H6 2E3yIuKJX4Yim3n
QG4hzAkhP-qVGIAjE1DufV0cz1gPME_qhQ7Ocl8F
Kw5ZUeyIZd6jkWAL1VU3Wby4-cMa_i5qsnXvyT1_vZ
OK3cVPouz4PauhKFdPoWK23QqCBGHGrmcyd3l9uwa
Oi6keWsjOn2ZNt9Qtk8m6A-Z9JyI4EKHjNKPbJm
FwGV6RuO4a4wIUMmg iqGN2yo6RaJgblN98ZR8.
W2puAOv6hH-gj4UnW-nPbt8N77BQoCFzQacHL3om
42E&dib_tag=se&keywords=Fantastic+mushrooms+-
+The+magical+world+at+our+feet&qid=1712212452&sbo
=RZvfv//HxDF%2BO5021pAnS A%3D%3D&sprefix=
fantastic+mushrooms+-+the+magical+world+at+our+feet
,aps,205&sr=8-2&linkCode=sl1&tag=tkpat-
21&linkId=2b18828cd05204019ac8c49191fc8a24&langu
age=de_DE&ref_=as_li_ss_tl

source references

https://tkp.at/2024/04/20/krebs-nach-impfung-am-vormarsch-was-dagegen-hilft/

https://tkp.at/2023/03/14/turbokrebs-nach-mrna-impfung-pfizer-kauft-firma-mit-krebs-medikament-um-43-milliarden-dollar/

https://www.dkfz.de/aktuelles/pressemitteilungen/detail/vitamin-d-supplementierung-moeglicher-gewinn-an-lebensjahren-bei-gleichzeitiger-kostenersparnis

https://www.pharmazeutische-zeitung.de/klassiker-im-neuen-licht/

https://www.drstrunz.de/aktuelles/2021/11/20211108_Vitamin_C_stoert_Chemotherapie.php

https://journals.plos.org/plosone/article?id=10.1371/journal.pone.0004592

https://tkp.at/2024/05/01/krebs-behandlung-hochwirksam-mit-chaga-heilpilz-studien/

https://pmc.ncbi.nlm.nih.gov/articles/PMC4946216/

https://pmc.ncbi.nlm.nih.gov/articles/PMC4946216/

https://www.frontiersin.org/journals/pharmacology/articles/10.3389/fphar.2023.1159516/full

https://www.frontiersin.org/journals/pharmacology/articles/10.3389/fphar.2023.1159516/full#B23

https://www.frontiersin.org/journals/pharmacology/articles/10.3389/fphar.2023.1159516/full#B23

https://www.frontiersin.org/journals/pharmacology/articles/10.3389/fphar.2023.1159516/full#B6

https://www.frontiersin.org/journals/pharmacology/articles/10.3389/fphar.2023.1159516/full#B8

https://www.frontiersin.org/journals/pharma-cology/articles/10.3389/fphar.2023.1159516/full#B5

https://www.frontiersin.org/journals/pharmacology/articles/10.3389/fphar.2023.1159516/full#B24

https://www.frontiersin.org/journals/pharmacology/articles/10.3389/fphar.2023.1159516/full#B43

https://www.frontiersin.org/journals/pharmacology/articles/10.3389/fphar.2023.1159516/full#B42

https://www.frontiersin.org/journals/pharmacology/articles/10.3389/fphar.2023.1159516/full#B7

https://www.fortunejournals.com/articles/huaier-effects-on-functional-compensation-with-destructive-ribosomal-rna-structure-after-antisarscov2-mrna-vaccination.html

https://www.fortunejournals.com/articles/huaier-effects-on-prevention-and-inhibition-of-spontaneous-sarscov2-virion-production-by-repeated-pfizerbiontech-mrna-vaccination.html

https://tkp.at/2023/05/30/japanische-studie-zeigt-wie-huaier-pilz-krebs-bekaempft-und-schaedliche-impf-spike-aus-dem-koerper-entfernt/
https://www.amazon.de/Huaier-Natural-Herb-Therapy-Cancer/dp/4991252504?&_encoding=UTF8&tag=tkpat-21&linkCode=ur2&linkId=c5c870926c3971a589b0e0ad42ceb05e&camp=1638&creative=6742

https://www.fortunejournals.com/articles/huaier-effects-on-prevention-and-inhibition-of-spontaneous-sarscov2-virion-production-by-repeated-pfizerbiontech-mrna-vaccination.html

https://tkp.at/2022/10/05/studie-c19-impfungen-fuehren-zu-vorzeitiger-zell-alterung-und-foerdern-krebserkrankung-video-mit-florian-schilling/

https://www.fortunejournals.com/articles/huaier-effects-on-functional-compensation-with-destructive-ribosomal-rna-structure-after-antisarscov2-mrna-vaccination.html

https://rumble.com/v1lz050-bad-news-from-japan.html

https://tkp.at/2024/05/08/schmetterlings-tramete-hilft-gegen-krebs-studien/

https://tkp.at/2025/02/09/die-starken-anti-krebs-wirkungen-von-pilzen/

https://petermcculloughmd.substack.com/p/the-remarkable-anti-cancer-potential?utm_source=post-email-title&publication_id=1119676&post_id=156696812&utm_campaign=email-post-title&isFreemail=false&r=8sqvf&triedRedirect=true&utm_medium=email

https://johncatanzaro.substack.com/cp/156522429

https://www.youtube.com/watch?v=0gIYQCjB_NU

https://www.sciencedirect.com/science/article/pii/S0753332222002906#bib141

https://pmc.ncbi.nlm.nih.gov/articles/PMC8483951/

https://pubmed.ncbi.nlm.nih.gov/36995535/

https://www.mdpi.com/1422-0067/24/5/4864

https://tkp.at/2024/12/18/tcm-medikament-huaier-pilz-laut-studien-hochwirksam-gegen-krebs-und-impfschaeden/

https://www.fortunejournals.com/articles/huaier-effects-on-prevention-and-inhibition-of-spontaneous-sarscov2-virion-production-by-repeated-pfizerbiontech-mrna-vaccination.html

https://pmc.ncbi.nlm.nih.gov/articles/PMC7737552/

https://www.spandidos-publications.com/10.3892/or.2015.3950

https://www.sciencedirect.com/science/article/abs/pii/S0378874124008778

https://tkp.at/2025/02/12/studie-aus-japan-starker-beleg-fuer-zusammenhang-von-krebs-und-mrna/

https://zenodo.org/records/14847943

https://alexberenson.substack.com/p/urgent-cancer-deaths-rose-in-japan?utm_source=post-email-title&publication_id=363080&post_id=156929538&utm_campaign=email-post-title&isFreemail=true&r=18rnaa&triedRedirect=true&utm_medium=email

https://tkp.at/2021/02/13/deutsche-krebsforscher-vitamin-d-schuetzt-vor-krebs-und-uebrigens-auch-vor-covid/

https://www.dkfz.de/aktuelles/pressemitteilungen/detail/vitamin-d-supplementierung-moeglicher-gewinn-an-lebensjahren-bei-gleichzeitiger-kostenersparnis

https://www.youtube.com/watch?v=JcZ2_8htKSw

https://www.youtube.com/watch?v=xEU7Hb8KrpM

https://tkp.at/2022/06/17/masken-koennten-das-wachstum-von-krebs-foerdern/

https://jamanetwork.com/journals/jamapediatrics/fullarticle/2781743

https://www.medrxiv.org/content/
10.1101/2022.05.10.22274813v1

https://www.mdpi.com/1660-4601/18/8/4344

https://journals.plos.org/plosone/article?id=10.1371/
journal.pone.0004592

https://tkp.at/2024/04/04/pilze-wirken-gegen-demenz-
und-staerken-das-immunsystem/
https://www.sciencedaily.com/releases/
2019/03/190312103702.htm

https://www.mayoclinic.org/diseases-conditions/mild-
cognitive-impairment/symptoms-causes/syc-20354578

https://www.nia.nih.gov/health/memory-loss-and-
forgetfulness/what-mild-cognitive-impairment

https://content.iospress.com/articles/journal-of-
alzheimers-disease/jad180959

https://www.verywellfit.com/mushroom-nutrition-facts-
calories-and-health-benefits-4117115

https://beatdepression.news/

https://febs.onlinelibrary.wiley.com/doi/10.1002/1873-
3468.14271

https://www.sciencedirect.com/science/article/abs/pii/
S0141813019304672

https://www.mdpi.com/2076-3921/10/9/1479

https://naturalpedia.com/colon-cancer-causes-side-effects-and-treatments-at-naturalpedia-com.html

https://www.sciencedirect.com/science/article/abs/pii/S0009279708004018?via%3Dihub

https://onlinelibrary.wiley.com/doi/10.1155/2018/5802634

https://www.mdpi.com/2304-8158/10/1/95

https://pubs.rsc.org/en/content/articlelanding/2019/ra/c9ra08245j

https://www.healthline.com/nutrition/reishi-mushroom-benefits

https://www.frontiersin.org/journals/aging-neuroscience/articles/10.3389/fnagi.2021.628860/full

https://translational-medicine.biomedcentral.com/articles/10.1186/s12967-021-02724-6

Link hierzu:
https://www.amazon.de/Fantastische-Pilze-magische-unseren-F%C3%BC%C3%9Fen/dp/B09K1T5YCW?__mk_de_DE=%C3%85M%C3%85%C5%BD%C3%95%C3%91&crid=BV7CXWHMMIRV&dib=eyJ2Ijoi MSJ9.5l9plfRLDRrzW1NmSe8H62E3yIuKJX4Yim3nQG4 hzAkhP-qVGIAjE1DufV0cz1gPME_qhQ7Ocl8FKw5ZUeyIZd6jkW AL1VU3Wby4-

cMa_i5qsnXvyT1_vZOK3cVPouz4PauhKFdPoWK23QqC
BGHGrmcyd3l9uwaOi6keWsjOn2ZNt9Qtk8m6A-
Z9JyI4EKHjNKPbJmFwGV6RuO4a4wIUMmgiqGN2yo6R
aJgblN98ZR8.W2puAOv6hH-gj4UnW-
nPbt8N77BQoCFzQacHL3om42E&dib_tag=se&keyword
s=Fantastische+Pilze+-
+Die+magische+Welt+zu+unseren+F%C3%BC
%C3%9Fen&qid=1712212452&sbo=RZvfv//HxDF
%2BO5021pAnSA%3D
%3D&sprefix=fantastische+pilze+-
+die+magische+welt+zu+unseren+f%C3%BC
%C3%9Fen,aps,205&sr=8-2&linkCode=sl1&tag=tkpat-
21&linkId=2b18828cd05204019ac8c49191fc8a24&langu
age=de_DE&ref_=as_li_ss_tl

https://tkp.at/2023/07/15/einschraenkungen-der-
verwendung-von-naturprodukten-fuer-heilung-und-
gesundheitsvorsorge/

https://nhppa.org/

https://www.efsa.europa.eu/de/topics/topic/novel-food

https://eur-lex.europa.eu/legal-content/DE/TXT/?
uri=CELEX:32015R2283

https://www.amazon.de/s?
k=schmetterlingstramete&language=de_DE&crid=MCAF
5RS11XU&linkCode=sl2&linkId=ba0b30f651e49e4e5a12
8f1eaf0399f1&sprefix=schmetterlingstramet%2Caps
%2C107&tag=tkpat-21&ref=as_li_ss_tl

https://www.amazon.de/s?
k=chaga+pilz&language=de_DE&crid=XAO2F82YLQGP
&linkCode=sl2&linkId=9f3d30e2dc62232f87f504952cb67
703&sprefix=chaga%2Caps%2C118&tag=tkpat-
21&ref=as_li_ss_tl

INFORMATION:

We make no warranty or accept any liability for the accuracy of the statements made in this book.